T0131671

Printed in the United States
by Baker & Taylor Publisher Services

PROSTATE CANCER SURVIVORS' ROADMAP

What to expect, treatment decisions + preparation + how to deal with recovery. Information and resources for Patients and Caregivers as they manage their Prostate Cancer journey.

PAUL SURFACE

PC Survivor & Advocate

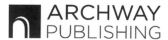

Archway Publishing books may be ordered through booksellers or by contacting:

Archway Publishing
1663 Liberty Drive
Bloomington, IN 47403
www.archwaypublishing.com
844-669-3957

ISBN: 978-1-6657-3105-8 (sc)
ISBN: 978-1-6657-3104-1 (hc)
ISBN: 978-1-6657-3106-5 (e)

Library of Congress Control Number: 2022918034

Print information available on the last page.

Archway Publishing rev. date: 10/25/2022

This book provides resources and support for patients and caregivers as they are faced with making decisions throughout their prostate cancer (PC) journeys. This book can help you learn

- where to find support and information for you PC decisions;
- what you can expect throughout your (PC) journey;
- what the PC journey process is like; and
- how PC will change your life.

It is important to realize that a Prostate Cancer Diagnosis is not an immediate death sentence. A PC Diagnosis will impact every aspect of a man's life and the lives of his family. Learn all you can, be your own advocate, and take life one day at a time. God bless.

Paul Surface PC Survivor & Advocate

Disclaimer: The prostate cancer information found in this book is a collection of tips and insights from fellow cancer survivors and from prostate cancer resources on various internet sites. All content shared by fellow cancer patient survivors reflects their experiences throughout their own cancer recovery processes.

This information is not qualified medical advice. Always seek the advice of your physician or other qualified health providers with any questions you may have regarding a medical condition.

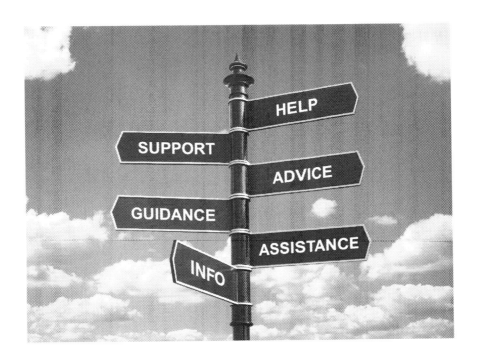

Note: Is there an easy way to connect to the URL links throughout the book? Yes, all URL'S provided can be accessed at https://www.prostateroadmap. com/ prostate-answers-articles-info. This will enable you to just click and read.

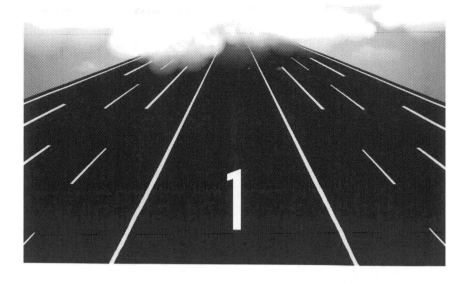

A PROSTATE CANCER
SURVIVOR'S PERSPECTIVE

You have been diagnosed with prostate cancer. Now what? Are you shocked, worried, confused, or looking for answers? What can you expect? A prostate cancer diagnosis is not an immediate death sentence. Will it change your life? Yes! No man expects a prostate cancer diagnosis. It's always a shock for both patients and families to hear the words, "You have cancer." The initial diagnosis and your prostate cancer journey will create highly stressful times. One of the biggest struggles for patients and families is dealing with the unknown.

This book was compiled to provide information for patients and caregivers as they make decisions throughout their prostate cancer journeys. You are not alone. When I was diagnosed, there was immediate shock, worry, and confusion. I had no knowledge regarding the world of prostate cancer. I was clueless and had no idea what a diagnosis would mean for my future. Prostate cancer diagnoses are common for men. One out of nine men receives a positive prostate diagnosis

during his lifetime. Prostate cancer is almost as common as breast cancer, which affects one in eight women. However, prostate cancer gets far less press coverage.

In the past, a cancer diagnosis was considered an immediate death sentence, but due to advancements in cancer medicine, there are multiple prostate cancer treatment options that allow millions of men to live long, productive lives. One of my doctors even called cancer a "chronic disease," because if the first treatment doesn't work, doctors can just try another option.

The prostate cancer journey can be as mentally and physically taxing for caregivers as it is for patients. Patients cannot do it alone. I wish there were definitive answers for the many questions that patients and caregivers need answered. No two patients are entirely alike, as responses to treatment can vary greatly. The personal recovery experience of each man will be impacted by age, health factors, treatment side effects, and the body's response to treatment. Two of the major factors for incontinence and sexual dysfunction after prostate cancer treatments are how much tissue was removed or damaged during the treatments and how far the cancer had spread.

My prostate cancer journey started in October of 2018, when my primary care doctor felt an asymmetric abnormality in my prostate gland during my yearly physical checkup. He recommended I see an oncologist, which I did in December of that year. Having no symptoms, pain, or discomfort before my diagnosis, I didn't immediately contact the oncologist. The oncologist performed tests and sent me to other prostate cancer specialists for additional opinions. At age seventy-one, I took a vacation from February through March of 2019 with

the doctor's blessing. The prostatectomy was performed in June of 2019. The decision to have a prostatectomy was easy, because my cancer had been deemed "aggressive." My doctor told me that he expected my cancer to return, but that hasn't happened yet.

A prostate cancer journey can be filled with unimaginable issues and challenges. Under highly stressful and debilitating circumstances, the patients and caregivers will make decisions that will impact their lives in major ways. Throughout my journey, I was constantly filled with stress from having to make multiple decisions. As is common with most men, I didn't want to contact my doctor or the medical community to ask questions. I turned to the internet to find direct, honest, and understandable information to help me make decisions. The internet provides many articles about prostate cancer by the medical community and advertisers, but that information did not answer my simple questions. I became frustrated by not finding answers that would help me make decisions. My frustration led me to compile resources and information from prostate cancer survivors to create this book, *Prostate Cancer Survivors' Roadmap,* and the website www.prostateroadmap. com. These were created to help patients and caregivers navigate and manage their prostate cancer journeys. I hope the doctors found your cancer early. I wish you and your family the best.

PC Survivor and Advocate P.S.

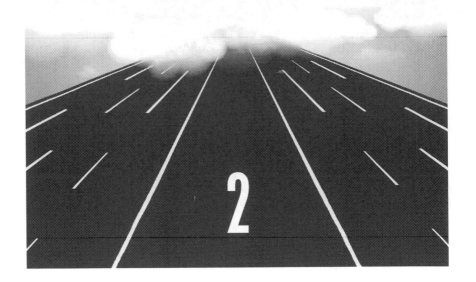

PROSTATE CANCER SURVIVOR LETTER FOR FRIENDS AND FAMILY

Being diagnosed with prostate, or any cancer, causes each of us and those connected to us, to handle the diagnosis in various ways. I have sent this very long 'letter' to family and friends in the past trusting it would help them to better understand how family and friends react. Feel free to save it and pass it on. "You have cancer!" Three little words that will change the lives of you and your family forever. It's terrifying. It's bewildering. It's overwhelming. It sucks. Cry a little. Cry a lot. But strive to get through the initial shock and emotional reaction as quickly as you can. You've got work to do. Don't bother trying to answer the question, "Why?" You'll spend too much energy to never get the answer. You'll need to focus that energy on what's ahead. Don't be ashamed that you have cancer. Have open and honest conversations about it with those around you; don't bottle it up. Find a tidbit of humor in the situation and inject it into the conversation. When you do, people will feel more comfortable around you.

Recognize, however, that some people will find being around cancer too difficult and will withdraw. Let them go, for their sake and yours. Most will return once they've had time to process what's happening. Relationships will be put to the test and may change. Remember that this isn't all about you. It's about those closest to you, too, and sometimes it can be more than they can bear. You'll have to be the strong one for them. Don't be surprised when some of your most casual acquaintances become your biggest supporters. Embrace them. Become your own advocate. Research, research, and research some more.

You may have the best medical team in the world, but question them. While they're highly trained medical professionals, they're still human. They may have their own self-interests in mind. If you ask a radiation oncologist what the best treatment option will be, he or she will likely say radiation. If you ask a surgeon, the answer will likely be surgery. You have to be comfortable with what's right for you, knowing all the potential risks, side effects, and complications.

When you go for your medical appointments, it is a good idea to take someone with you as you won't remember all that is said. Make a list of questions to appointments and take notes of the answers. With the permission of the doctor possibly they would allow you to record the appointment. Anything that will help you remember all the information given to you is important. Seek out other patients who have had your cancer, whether a friend, a family member, or in a support group (or even through a blog). They can be the greatest resource available to you. They can tell you their first-hand experience and how the cancer and the treatment impacted their daily life. Recognize that each case is unique, so take their input with a grain of salt and realize you may not have the same result.

You can research and consult with your medical team until the cows come home, but at some point you're going to have to make a decision. You. It's your body and your life. You have to be comfortable that your research was thorough, and that you'll make the best decision possible with the information at hand at that point in time. Then place your trust in your medical team to do the best they can. You will be stressed. You'll have "cancer" on the mind 24/7. Figure out ways to distract yourself from the cancer thoughts even for a few hours. Go to a movie, take a drive through the country, take a hike—whatever works for you. The stress can wear you down physically. Get plenty of rest after those sleepless nights; watch your nutrition; get some exercise. You've got to be as healthy as you can going into the challenges ahead. All of this is far easier said than done. I know.

Friends and family will offer assistance; take them up on their offers. They're not there to pity you; they're there to offer genuine help and support. Don't let pride get in the way. While we all hope for the best possible outcome, the harsh reality is that not everyone survives cancer. Make sure your affairs are in order, especially advanced medical directives, and that your family understands and will honor your desires.

Being told you have cancer is not the end; it's the beginning of a process. If you are diagnosed with early-stage cancer, the diagnosis is the beginning of your process to determine what treatment option is best for you. But even if you are diagnosed with late-stage cancer, and are considered to be terminal, it's still the beginning of the process to figure out the best options for your remaining time.

Lastly, even if your cancer allows for successful treatment, cancer will always be in your thoughts long after the treatment ends. A little "recurrence cloud" will follow you around every day, as you wonder whether or not the cancer will return. Once you introduce cancer into your vocabulary, it's there for good, whether the actual disease is there or not. I wish you and your family all the best as you begin your own journey.

PC Survivor C. S.

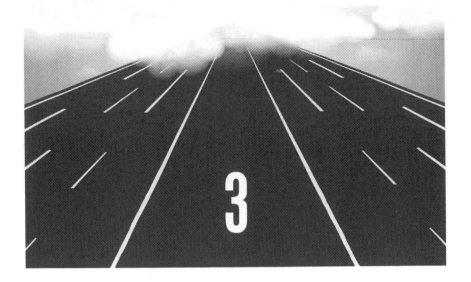

THE PROSTATE CANCER
JOURNEY'S FOUR STAGES

What is the prostate cancer diagnosis and journey process? Once a patient is diagnosed, there are four stages: diagnosis, decision, treatment, and home recovery (DIY). The diagnosis stage includes tests and second opinions. During the decision stage, the patient and caregiver choose a treatment procedure. The best way to describe the treatment stage and the home recovery stage is to use the analogy of a long-distance stage race. During the treatment stage, the race car is driven by a professional driver (the doctor) who carefully follows a precisely designed protocol map and is supported by a highly trained professional team. During this stage, the patient is riding in the back seat. Most prostate cancer survivors voice how easy the treatment stage is compared to the recovery stage. During the home recovery stage of the race, the race car is no longer a race car. It's a fixer-upper. The car is driven by an impaired patient with treatment side effects and who is possibly heavily medicated. There are no designed protocol maps to follow, and the support team has no training!

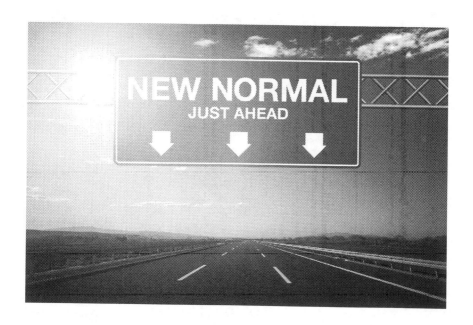

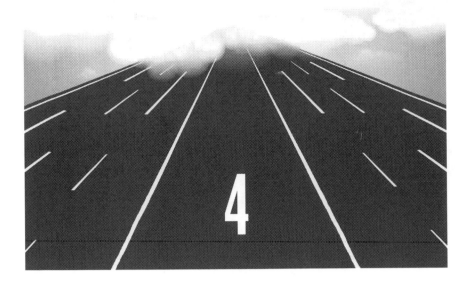

THE PATIENT'S NEW NORMAL LIFE

- How will our life change post treatment?
- What should you expect?

Overview

Each man's recovery journey is different, depending on treatment chosen, cancer stage, and the body's reaction to treatment.

After prostate cancer treatments, the patient's *normal* daily living activities will become *abnormal* daily living activities. For my three-month post-surgery checkup, I prepared a long list of the issues and challenges I faced that worried me during my first weeks of recovery. I considered them to be abnormal experiences. I shared this list with my doctor, expecting some level of concern. However, he waived each item off as if the issues were expected. All the issues I considered to be abnormal were considered totally normal and routine to the medical community. *Normal?* The issues and challenges were absolutely *abnormal* to me!

If you are wondering if all patients have abnormal experiences similar to those of other prostate patients after treatments, the answer is yes. While most men experience minimal issues after treatments, some men may find that the *abnormals* may become their *new normals* for months or years to come. Becoming knowledgeable about the issues and challenges you will face, setting realistic expectations with yourself, and being patient from the outset throughout your recovery journey are musts.

Resources: Patient's New Normal

- **Anyone Been There and Done That?**
  https://www.cancerresearchuk.org/about-cancer/cancer-chat/thread/prostate-cancer-anyone-been-there-done-that
- **The Long, Wet Road Back to Normal**
  https://www.pcf.org/c/long-wet-road-back-normal/
- **I Reject the Notion I'm on a Cancer Journey**
  https://www.cancer.net/blog/2017-10/i-reject-notion-im-cancer-journey

- Additional PC information provided in Chapter 20: PC Resources.

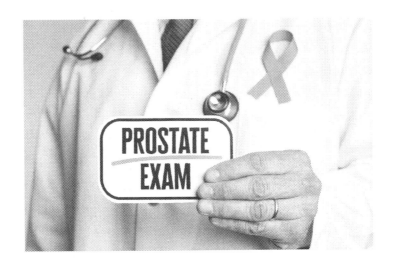

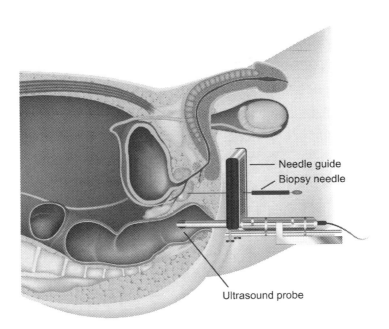

Needle guide
Biopsy needle
Ultrasound probe

Prostate biopsy

Paul Surface

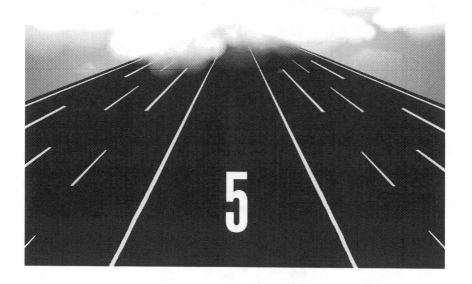

DIAGNOSIS STAGE

- Yikes, I have cancer!

Overview

It's always a shock to hear the words "you have cancer," both for patients and families. One of the biggest struggles of having a prostate cancer diagnosis is dealing with the unknown.

A prostate cancer diagnosis is not an immediate death sentence! Prostate cancer is recognized to be a slow-growing cancer. Oncology teams have a relaxed attitude relating to a PC diagnosis and do not seem to be in a hurry. Doctors don't seem to panic, but it is quite scary for those of us who have been diagnosed with prostate cancer.

How does a man know he has prostate cancer? PC is like most other cancers—there are no or minimal signs pointing to the existence of cancer. The only way to confirm the cancer exists is through medical tests and exams.

Survivor Story

Age: 59; Treatment: Radiation; Gleason score: 10

When I was diagnosed in October 2014. I had Stage 4 metastatic diagnosed with PC and given 6 months to live! Thankfully, that was 7 years ago! The cancer had spread to my spine. Since it had already spread to my bones there was no need to remove the prostate, hence no surgery I had 10 rounds of radiation on my spine and left femur, followed by 6 rounds of chemo. I have been getting Lupron injections since I was diagnosed. However, I think your project is valuable. I think all cancer patients wish they had more access to "inside" information. As we know, doctors don't always tell the whole story, or at least not the parts we want to hear about. Don't let the bastards get you down! I wish you continued success in your recovery. My wife tells me it's now time to stop talking about my death.

PC Survivor and Friend M. H.

The Prostate Cancer Diagnosis Process

Rectal Exam: A rectal examination of the prostate gland should be part of a man's yearly physical. The doctor will feel the prostate gland to ascertain any abnormalities. My doctor found mine to be asymmetric and sent me to an oncologist.

PSA Test: A PSA blood test is used to diagnosis the potential existence of cancer in a man's prostate gland. A high reading indicates the possibility of cancer.

Biopsy: A biopsy of the prostate gland is performed to determine the actual existence and extent of cancer. From the results of the biopsy, a Gleason score and cancer stage is assigned for the level of cancer in the prostate gland. If a patient is given a high Gleason score, the high-level score does not necessarily equate to the level of treatment success a patient will experience.

Your medical team will analyze the PSA test and biopsy results to make next step recommendations. The PSA test and biopsy do not provide information regarding the spread of cancer outside of the prostate gland. The two ways to confirm cancer has spread throughout the man's body is either during prostate surgery or by using imaging scans.

MRI or CT Scan: Imaging scans can be ordered by the doctor to:

- Find cancer spread in the body;
- Determine stage of cancer;
- Help plan need for non-surgical treatment;
- Show if tumor has changed; and/or
- Determine if the cancer has returned after treatment.

There is a lot of conflicting advice about the age a man should have the PSA test. No matter what the doctor says, the

PSA test needs to be part of a man's regular physical exam. It's your life, so be your own advocate! Ask your doctor to add the PSA component to your blood draw.

Resources: Diagnosis Stage

- **Getting a second opinion**
  https://news.cancerconnect.com/newly-diagnosed/the-importance-of-getting-a-second-opinion
- **Early detection screening for PC**
  https://news.cancerconnect.com/prostate-cancer/psa-early-detection-screening-prevention-of-prostate-cancer
- **Importance of getting a PSA**
  https://www.urologyspecialistsnc.com/importance-getting-psa-screening/
- **What to know in detail about PC**
  https://www.medicalnewstoday.com/articles/150086.php
- **Prostate Cancer and You podcast**
  https://masspcc.org › page › podcast
- **What happens after a prostate cancer diagnosis (YouTube)**
  https://www.youtube.com/watch?v=nY0jYIj4r1I

- Additional PC information provided in Chapter 20: PC Resources.

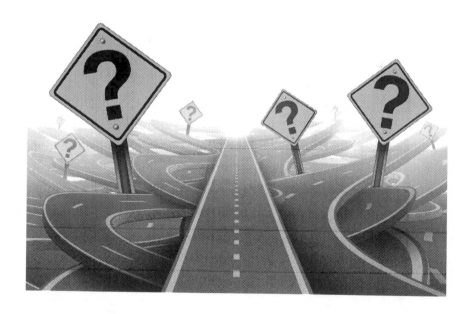

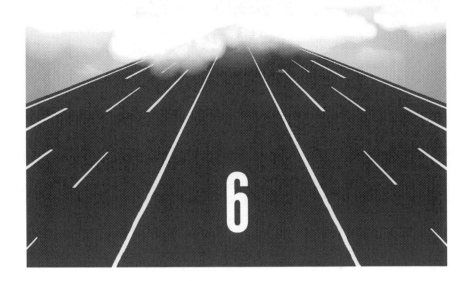

DECISION STAGE

- How do you choose the best PC treatment for your cancer?

Overview

Making your treatment decision can be the most stressful part of a PC journey. Patients and caregivers are challenged because of their lack of knowledge and being faced with a total unknown. Medical teams perform a variety of tests and analyze the reports to be able to recommend a treatment approach. Typically, a doctor will recommend the treatment that is his or her specialty, so it is important to get a second opinion from doctors of different specialties. My doctor told me I owed it to myself to get a second opinion. I cannot express strongly enough the need for a patient to get a *second opinion*. Make sure you thoroughly understand the pros, cons, and side effects of each procedure. It all comes down to doing the PC research and choosing the option and medical team that seems most comfortable for you and your caregivers. It is your life and future! The bottom line is that each patient needs to be his own advocate.

I wish there were definitive answers for all of the many questions a patient and caregiver needs to have answered as they face the many issues and challenges throughout the PC journeys. The PSA level and Gleason score are cancer indicators for diagnosis, but a high reading does *not* necessarily equate to the level of success from treatments. No two patients are entirely alike, as treatment and responses to treatment can vary greatly. The personal recovery experience will be impacted by treatment choice, age, any additional health factors, the treatment side effects, and the body's response to treatment. One of the major factors for incontinence and sexual dysfunction after PC treatment depends on how much tissue is removed or damaged during the treatments.

Treatment Options to Consider

- **Active Surveillance Option**: wait and see
- **Surgical Option**: traditional surgery or robotic surgery
- **Non-Surgical Options**:
    - hormone therapy
    - radiation therapy (radiotherapy)
    - chemotherapy
    - immunotherapy
- Additional PC information provided in Chapter 20: PC Resources.

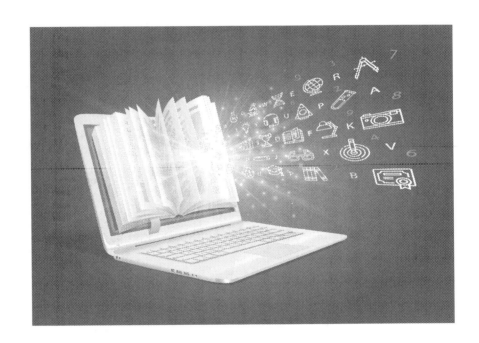

Paul Surface

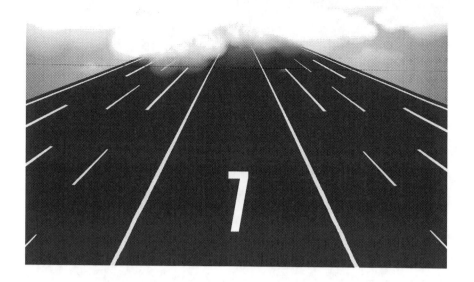

TREATMENT PROCEDURE CHOICES

- What is the best PC treatment for the patient?

Overview

The prostate cancer research community has spent years researching and developing treatment options for prostate cancer. A prostate cancer diagnosis is not necessarily an immediate death sentence.

> **Active Surveillance:** Some men will receive the recommendation for active surveillance. This means waiting to see what happens. While this may be sound advice, a patient needs to be his own advocate, get a second opinion, and weigh all the pros and cons for moving forward with a PC treatment procedure or active surveillance.

Surgical Options: This could be either traditional surgery or robotic surgery. If the choice is surgery, a patient can be somewhat self-sufficient, as long as he prepares the home, knows what to expect, and prepares for it.

- **Traditional Surgery**: This is an invasive procedure as the surgeon removes the entire prostate gland, the seminal vesicles, and some surrounding tissue, if necessary, not using the assistance of advanced surgical technology.
- **Robotic Prostatectomy**: A minimally invasive procedure using the assistance of advanced surgical technology.

Resources: Surgical Options

- **YouTube: Surgery or Radiotherapy**
  https://www.youtube.com/watch?v=CAmOAeRQ0Ps

- **YouTube: Robotic Surgery for Prostate Cancer**
  https://www.youtube.com/watch?v=4gqWir1Ja5g

- Additional PC information provided in Chapter 20: PC Resources.

Resources: Non-Surgical Options

Each non-surgical treatment creates a wide variety of issues and side effects.

- **Hormone Therapy**: This is also called androgen suppression therapy. It removes, blocks, or adds hormones to treat prostate cancer. The goal is to reduce levels of male hormones, called androgens, in the body to stop them from fueling prostate cancer cells.
  - **YouTube: Hormone and Chemotherapy** https://www.youtube.com/watch?v=Yq1Rr3R6UsM
- **Radiation Therapy**: This is also called X-ray therapy. It involves the use of high-energy beams or radioactive seeds to eliminate tumors. High levels of radiation are used to kill prostate cancer cells or keep them from growing and dividing, while minimizing damage to healthy cells.
  - **YouTube: Radiation Therapy for PC** https://www.youtube.com/watch?v=goyTxNuMCho
  - **YouTube: Surgery or Radiotherapy** https://www.youtube.com/watch?v=CAmOAeRQ0Ps
- **Chemotherapy**: is the use of any one or combination of cancer-fighting drugs. It is prescribed in cases of recurrent or advanced prostate cancer that has not responded to hormone treatment. It is not used to treat early-stage disease, except as part of a clinical trial.

- **Immunotherapy**: uses a person's own immune system to fight the cancer by changing how the immune system works so it can find and attack cancer cells.
  - **YouTube Prostate Cancer Immunotherapy Stories**
    https://www.youtube.com/watch?v=uaa3RUVfTOg
- Additional PC information provided in Chapter 20: PC Resources.

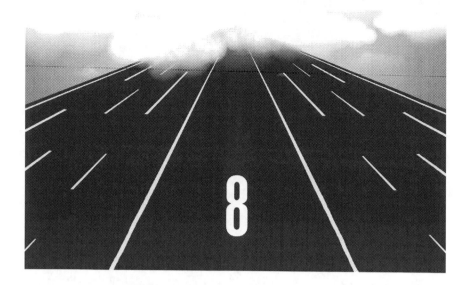

MANAGING THE HOME RECOVERY (DIY) STAGE

- You are home for recovery after your treatment(s). Now what?

Overview

What I call do-it-yourself (DIY) home recovery starts as soon as the patient gets home after treatment(s). The patient and caregivers will be making all of the recovery decisions, both big and small. Home recovery can create a great deal of stress, due to lack of knowledge and skills needed to manage the types of challenges and issues that will be faced. What issues will you need to manage? Insights and tips can be found in this book from prostate cancer survivors, as they share the personal experiences of their PC journeys. Find help in the Catheter Management and Recovery Issues, Challenges, Side-Effects sections.

Insights and Tips:

A patient can be somewhat self-sufficient, as long as he knows what to expect and prepare for it. As a prostate cancer patient, I was so preoccupied with the idea of having *cancer* and making sure I followed the directions for surgery, I spent no time contemplating issues I might face during recovery at home. Once home, it immediately became necessary to make decisions regarding the issues and challenges I was facing. This was in addition to being handicapped with post-surgery trauma, a catheter bag, and lingering effects of anesthesia. I was woefully unprepared. It wasn't pretty.

General/Household Tips:

— Identify where to hang catheter while taking a shower
— Identify where to hang catheter at bedside
— Establish a Kegel exercise routine
— Make a contact list of your support team
— Stock food: pre-cooked meals, microwavable items
— Safety check: rugs, electric cords, stairs
— Accessibility: dishes, glasses, refrigerator
— Pay bills/arrange finances
— Update will and health care proxy

Resources: Home Recovery Stage

- **How the Body Heals Itself after Surgery**
  https://www.glenviewterrace.com/blog/six-ways-to-speed-up-the-healing-process-after-surgery/

- **Quality Outline: Discharge instructions**
  https://www.hopkinsmedicine.org/brady-urology-institute/patient-information/_docs/dr.handischarge_instructions.pdf
- **What to Expect at Home: Icing after surgery**
  https://myhealth.alberta.ca/Health/aftercareinformation/pages/conditions.aspx?hwid=ud2576
- **Going Home After Robotic Surgery**
  http://urology.iupui.edu/img/pdfs/prostiurobothome06.pdf
- **After a Prostatectomy: Post Operative Care**
  http://www.urology.uci.edu/prostate/Postop.html
- **Blog: Recovery Insights**
  https://www.google.com/search?q=home+recovery+after+surgery+blog&ie=UTF-8&oe=UTF-8&hl=en-us&client=safari

- Additional PC information provided in Chapter 20: PC Resources.

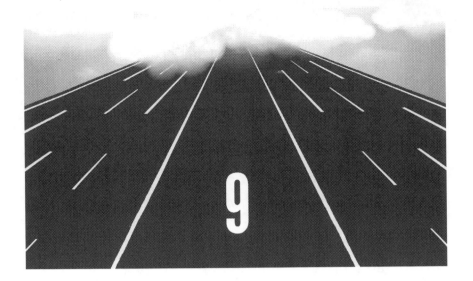

CATHETER MANAGEMENT TIPS AND INSIGHTS

- What challenges and issues will the patient face with an inserted catheter?

Overview

A catheter will be inserted during your surgery. Some men need to leave the inserted catheter in place for weeks. Wearing a catheter creates a range of logistical issues and challenges that will result in different levels of pain and frustration for patients. The pain and frustration can be mitigated by establishing a plan of action for showering, walking, lying down, eating, sleeping and, if you find it comfortable enough, sitting.

Tips and Insights

- **Securing the Catheter to Your Body:** To minimize issues, you will need to make sure the catheter hose is secure and stable on your leg. The patches will be placed on your leg without taking your anatomy into account. You may decide that the catheter would be more comfortable and secure by being placed higher, lower, or on your other leg. There is no problem making the change, as long as it is secure. Be especially aware of the hose and/or patch coming loose when changing your clothes or moving around, and especially when walking.
- **Catheter Flow:** The catheter is constructed to always flow into the bag. *As long as* the bag is below your body and hose is not crimped, there will be no problem. The hose can even be in a U shape.

Survivor Story

I had surgery on a Tuesday, spent night in hospital. On Saturday I went to a soccer game with urine bag strapped to my leg under loose clothes. Catheter removed the following Tuesday of [*sic*] doctor's office.

PC Survivor and Friend D. W.

Bedside Set-Up: Set up and secure the hose and bag for safety to make sure there is no accidental tripping or pulling when you roll over while sleeping. There are three criteria to make sure that urine will flow to the bag properly when you are in bed.

- The bag must be below the body position.
- The bag cannot lay directly on the floor. Putting it in a waste bin or bucket will stabilize it.
- The hose cannot be crimped.

I obsessed about the catheter and put together an elaborate configuration to have the catheter hose go from my body, to a chair, and angled down to a bucket. It is not necessary, as the three components above are all you need.

Stabilizing the Catheter and Hose: It is important to stabilize the hose for safety. Flow can become restricted if the hose becomes crimped, which can result in a dangerous back flow of urine. The cord itself can also become a trip hazard. Consider using Velcro strips to attach it to an anchor, such as a small table, chair, or bed stand, or the bucket. This will allow you to easily detach the hose from the anchor when moving from one location to another.

Maintaining Hygiene: Having absorbent pads, old rags, sanitary wipes, paper towels, and Kleenex available at all times is critical, especially throughout the journey. Even with the catheter in, urine will often dribble when you lie down or stand up. You should be prepared to deal with clean-up when getting out of bed, standing after sitting, standing after having a bowel movement, or when brushing your teeth or eating. The prostateroadmap.com website provides the Home Recovery checklist and Home Recovery Needs Store with items you will need (available at https://www.prostateroadmap.com/prostate-home-recovery-needs-store).

- Keeping your body and floors clean is vital.
- Be prepared to shower multiple times a day for the first few weeks. It does not need to be a complete shower. Information is at the prostateroadmap.com website.
- Using healing antibiotic ointment and salve ointment on the penis tip throughout the day will help to mitigate chafing.
- Do not use antibiotic ointment or salve ointment on your stitches.
- Make sure the bag's empty spout is directly over toilet bowl when emptying your urine bag.
- You will need to empty the urine bag every few hours during the night.
- You may need to empty the urine bag during your walk so that it will not back flow.

Sitting Pain: *Ouch!* The catheter tube was inserted during the surgery and is most likely a Foley catheter. The catheter tube passes from the bladder through the end of your penis and into a catheter bag. One area the hose passes over is the perineum, basically the floor of your torso between your legs. I was not aware of the perineum before the surgery, but I became quite aware of it during recovery. The catheter tube presses directly against the perineum when you sit (or attempt to sit), causing a great deal of pressure to an already tender spot. Whether sitting in a hard or soft chair, sitting up straight, at an angle, on a pillow, on a donut pillow, or on a stool, you can expect to be uncomfortable.

You may find your best option is to transition between lying down and standing. I was unable to sit for the entire time the catheter was in as the pain became worse each day. Even after the catheter was removed, I experienced residual sitting pain for three weeks. *It hurts!*

Penis Tip: The tip of the penis can become tender and irritated from movement, due to the gravitational pull on the tube. Using healing antibiotic ointments, salve ointments, and pain relief medicine ointments can help you manage the irritation.

Slippage When Changing Clothes: If you are not careful and the bag slips down, you will experience a major pull on your penis.

Dressing: Putting on clothes while wearing a catheter needs to be approached with care. Slip the catheter bag from the top of your pants/underwear down through the corresponding leg as the leg strap is attached.

Sleeping: You may find it more comfortable to be in a bed, on a sofa, or in a reclining chair, but get used to sleeping on your back, or on one side, until the catheter is removed. Some patients indicate they were able sleep on their stomachs. A knee pad and wedge pillow can help. A reclining chair has been recommended as a great option for sleeping.

Dribble and Bowel Movement: Expect dribble from the catheter tube/ penis area during and after bowel movements. Have paper towels readily available for the floor and for self-cleaning.

Bowel Movement: It will take from four to six days after surgery until your body is ready to allow you to have a bowel movement. The first and second bowel movements will most likely be hard as rocks. *Make sure to take stool softeners daily.* Bowel movements will get easier after a while. You may experience a watery stool a few times, but this is nothing to worry about.

Walking and Catheter Support: Walking with a catheter can be a significant challenge. Make sure the catheter tube does not move around and tug on the end of your penis during walking. The catheter tube was most likely attached to your leg. You may want to change the strap onto your thigh to make it easier to walk. It is okay to move the catheter to different parts of your leg.

The catheter tube support you received from the hospital may not be adequate for your walks. You may need to provide additional support by securing the tube with Velcro strips and/or an ACE bandage to help support the tube. You can also purchase a heavy-duty catheter tube support at https://www.prostateroadmap.com/prostate-home-recovery-needs-store.

- Make sure the tube is strapped securely on your body.
- Place the catheter bag into an over the shoulder bag when walking outside.
- Intermittently check how much urine has collected in the tube during your walk. If the hose is too full, lift up the hose to have the urine flow into the bag.

I did not have any information on how to stabilize my catheter. I tried using adhesive tape, but that didn't work. I even attached a string as a shoulder strap onto the hose just under the lowest hose regulator valve to limit gravitational pulling down of the tube on my penis. Nope, that didn't really work. You definitely don't need to go the string route. A heavy duty catheter hose strap, Velcro strips, or ACE bandage will do the trick. Walking as soon as possible will speed up your healing process. Don't forget: *short walks count!*

Urine Bottle and Bed Pad: The reusable urine bottle and

a bed pad are a must after catheter is removed. (Recovery items are available at https://www.prostateroadmap.com/prostate-home-recovery-needs-store.)

Resources: Catheter Management

- **Articles on Managing a Catheter at Prostateroadmap. com** https://www.prostateroadmap.com/prostate-answers-articles-info
- **Foley Catheter Placement and Care** https://www.drugs.com/cg/foley-catheter-placement-and-care.html has a medically reviewed article with clear and succinct information on the Foley catheter, managing the equipment, and how to handle issues that may come up.
- **Foley Catheter: Home Instructions** https://intermountainhealthcare.org/ext/Dcmnt?ncid=520589057 is a helpful fact sheet for patients and caregivers from Intermountain Healthcare.
- **Urine Drainage Bag and Leg Bag Care** https://my.clevelandclinic.org/health/articles/14832-urine-drainage-bag-and-leg-bag-care describes the process for attaching, removing, and cleaning urine drainage and leg bags.
- **Tips for Holding your Catheter in Place** https://livingwithacatheter.com/tips-for-holding-your-catheter-in-place/ is just one valuable post from Livingwithacatheter.com that may make your catheter experience more manageable. There's also a forum

on this site and a series of articles that you may find helpful.

- **Sleeping with a Catheter**
  https://www.google.com/search?q=tips+on+ways+to+set+up+catheter+for+bedside+use&ie=UTF-8&oe=UTF-8&hl=en-us&client=safari

- **Troubleshooting Your Catheter**
  https://www.healthywa.wa.gov.au/Articles/ST/Troubleshooting-for-your-catheter offers good catheter management information from the Western Australian Department of Health.

- **Catheter Care Steps: Urinary Catheter Care for Caregivers**
  https://elizz.com/caregiver-resources/urinary-catheter-care-for-caregivers/ is for caregivers supporting a patient with a urinary catheter. This article provides catheter care tips that will help reduce the risk of problems, and it highlight concerns that may need assessment by the patient's health care provider.

- Additional PC information provided in Chapter 20: PC Resources

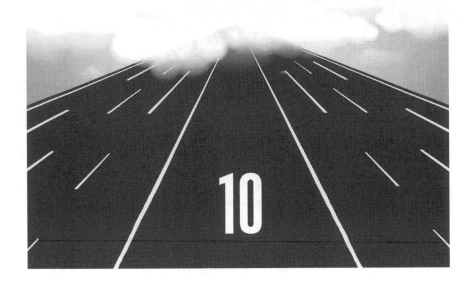

RECOVERY ISSUES, CHALLENGES, AND SIDE EFFECTS

- What can the patient expect after PC treatment procedures?

Overview

Once the catheter is removed, the patient should expect his bowel, peeing, and/or penile function to be compromised at various levels. Most likely, the bowel dysfunction will return to normal relatively quickly in four to six days. The penile and peeing dysfunction are typically the most significant challenges a prostate cancer patient will face during hisr recovery. Most literature indicates it may take up to one year to gain full control of your peeing and penile functions, while some patients may never fully recover.

Recovery Tips and Insights

For some men, recovery is not a problem. After surgery or non-surgery treatments, the patient needs to keep walking, not overdo, and drink lots of liquids. As for sex and intimacy, many men worry about having sexual dysfunction and the inability to have an erection. Will the inability to have an erection be the end of a healthy sex life? No! A man can still experience sexual desire, feelings, and emotions, and be capable of intimacy with a supportive partner, including a sense of climax. The climax does not go away, only no semen comes out. Some men find the climax and sexual intimacy experience to be as intense, or possibly more intense, than before the surgery.

Must Reads:

- Voiding after catheter removal, urinating after the catheter is removed. Talk to your medical team.
- Home Recovery Needs Checklist: this list of recovery items is available as a PDF download at https://www.prostateroadmap.com/prostate-homerecovery-needs-list.

Catheter Removal/Extraction Day

Many men ask, "Does the catheter removal hurt?" No, but thinking about it hurts more than the actual removal. The removal of the catheter doesn't hurt, but the thought of it does. The mental anxiety regarding the catheter removal is the same anxiety a man can feel about jumping into freezing water or into a hot spa. Just breathe and relax.

Voiding

I cannot stress strongly enough that you need to be aware of the word *voiding*. I was quite perplexed regarding the actual definition for *voiding*. The issue of *voiding* has the potential to cause a great deal of stress. Immediately after catheter removal, the medical team will give the patient instructions that he must *void* within six to twelve hours after the catheter is removed. The *voiding* indicates the patient is capable of passing urine. *If* the patient does not *void*, the medical team instructs the patient to return and have the catheter re-inserted. *Yikes!* The thought of having the catheter re-inserted caused a great deal of anxiety.

> FYI: How did I handle voiding? Did I call the medical team to report that I was having issues? No I did not, because there was no-way I wanted to have the catheter re-inserted. So I opted for definition B. below.

Voiding Definition (multiple choice): What does it mean to *void*?

A. Standing at a toilet and emitting a long stream, short stream, or dribble of urine; or
B. Dribbling urine into two to six diapers within the first six to twelve hours.

Answer: Both of the above.

I chose option B, figuring urine was definitely flowing. After a few weeks, I was able to meet option A. No harm, no foul! To be clear, make sure you discuss *voiding* with your medical team and ask them to be specific about *voiding*.

Hygiene

Ongoing efforts to maintain good hygiene and the use of adult diapers/guards will be necessary to keep your living space clean and yourself healthy during recovery. Having rags or towels on hand at all times will be critical. Here are some additional hygiene tips.

- Keep genitals clean and dry.
- Keep bedroom and bathroom floors clean by using mats and clothes or towels on floor.
- Keep bed clean with a mat and cover it with a towel, as the mat generates a lot of heat.
- Keep toilet and sink clean.
- Clean shower area as necessary.
- Use baby powder liberally.
- Use ointments when necessary.
- Change out rags and towels daily.

Absorbent Guards or Diapers

There are two options for protection from leakage. The use of an absorbent guard or diaper is for leakage protection. The need to protect against bowel issues is not really a factor with PC, so the diaper is not necessary. Diapers can be the option immediately after the catheter is removed, due to the amount of potential leakage. The problem with diapers is that they generate a great deal of heat. The combination of leakage and a humid diaper can lead to a yeast infection.

During the night, after the leakage subsided and there was some level of control when lying down, I decided I did not need either the absorbent guard or diaper. I just used a soft rag in my shorts. You may find that guards may be a better option during the day. Expect to use six to nine diapers and/ or guards per day for one week after the catheter is removed, at a minimum.

> **WARNING:** The combination of leakage and a humid diaper can lead to a yeast infection. Www. prostateoadmap.com provides additional information.

Underwear and Jockstrap

You will need to use brief underwear or a jockstrap to hold the absorbent guards in place.

Pain! Pain! Pain! in the Perineum Area

Sitting pain from the inserted catheter tube can be a major problem. While the catheter was in place, sitting was basically impossible. The pain in the perineum area continued to be uncomfortable and painful. Even after the catheter was removed, there was pain. By the fourth week after removal, I could finally sit for an hour.

What if you need to use your computer when it hurts to sit?

I used a large box on a table as a computer stand. Finally, I decided to purchase a computer stand. Computer stands are available for purchase at https://www.prostateroadmap.com/prostate-home-recovery-needs-storeoffers.

Sharp Pain/Nerve Regeneration

Most patients report minimal sensitivity in the surgical area for the first couple of weeks, until the nerve endings start the regeneration process.

Bam! A shooting pain! The regenerating nerve endings would throw in a few sharp jolts of pain every now and again to remind me they were doing their job. It started as a feeling/sensation of something going on in my lower abdomen/genital area. Over the next few weeks, the area became more sensitive and I experienced minor pain and discomfort.

Stomach and Stitches

For most patients, there is no significant pain in the stomach or from the stitches. While the stomach muscles typically tighten up after surgery, they will gradually loosen over the next few weeks. Expect the stitches to be inflamed, and you may have a bloated stomach.

To mitigate heat generated by the stitches, you can use ice packs liberally throughout the process. Do not use lubricating ointment on the stitches, unless your medical provider recommends otherwise.

Kegels

My medical team did not bring up the need to do Kegels before my surgery. I found out post-surgery and I wish I had been told. My yoga teacher said to prevent incontinence and strengthen the pelvic muscles, imagine that your pelvic muscles are a tent and try to pick up the tent from the top.

Resources: Kegels

- **Kegel Exercises**
  https://www.mayoclinic.org/healthy-lifestyle/mens-health/in-depth/kegel-exercises-for-men/art-20045074
- **Kegels for Men**
  https://www.medicinenet.com/kegel_exercises_for_men/article.htm
- **Kegels for Men In-Depth**
  https://www.wikihow.fitness/Do-Kegel-Exercises-for-Men
- **Kegel Insights**
  https://comments.medicinenet.com/kegel_exercises_for_men/patient-comments-4091.htm
- **Living With Incontinence and Value of Kegels**
  https://well.blogs.nytimes.com/2009/03/03/living-with-incontinence-after-prostate-cancer/
- **Kegel Exercises After Prostate Surgery** on YouTube

- Additional PC information provided in Chapter 20: PC Resources.

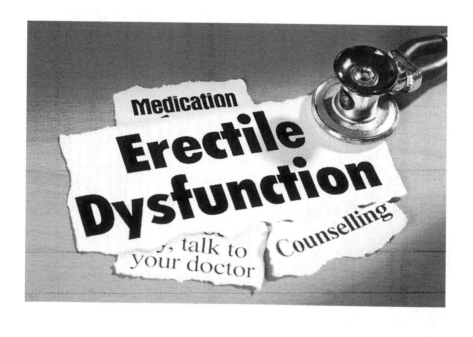

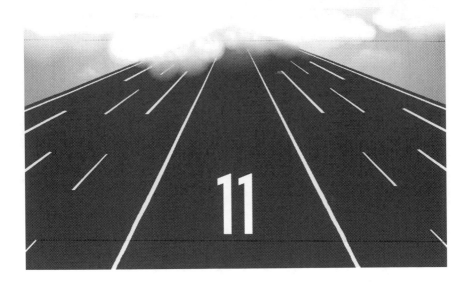

DYSFUNCTION CHALLENGES
AND ISSUES

- What dysfunction challenges and issues will a man experience after PC treatment?
- Survivors share their Dysfunction experiences and ways to manage peeing, bowel, and sexual dysfunction post-treatment.

Overview

Once the catheter is removed, the ability for you to resume normal bladder (peeing), bowel, and sexual function will most likely be compromised. The treatment(s) create dysfunction. Resuming control is often the *most significant* obstacle for prostate cancer treatment survivors to manage during recovery. Most literature indicates it may take up to one year to gain full control of your bladder or sexual function after surgery. Some men never regain control.

There is *no way* a patient will not have *dysfunction* after

PC treatment procedures, as the prostate gland is in close proximity to multiple other organs (bladder, urinary gland, sexual glands, bowel tracks, localized nerves, and muscles). After prostate cancer procedures, the patient will need to manage the *absolutely abnormal*.

Once the catheter is removed, a patient should *expect* his bladder, bowel, and/or sexual function to be compromised. I was totally blindsided with all of the post treatment issues and challenges that were the direct result of my prostatectomy. All diagnosed patients and fellow prostate cancer survivors experience some level of *dysfunction*, whether they have surgical or non-surgical treatment procedures.

The bladder (peeing) and penile dysfunction are the most significant obstacles prostate cancer patients will face during their recovery. The bowel dysfunction will return to normal relatively quickly

Bowel Dysfunction

Solid waste that is excreted from the body moves slowly down the intestines, and under normal circumstances, the resultant stool exits through the rectum and then the anus. Damage to the rectum can result in bowel problems, including rectal bleeding, diarrhea, or urgency.

After a prostatectomy, it is very rare (less than 1 percent) for men to have altered bowel function after surgery. In rare cases of locally advanced prostate cancer where the cancer has invaded the rectum, surgery may result in rectal damage.

Resources: Bowel **Dysfunction**

- **Bowel Dysfunction Side Effects**
  https://www.pcf.org/about-prostate-cancer/prostate-cancer-side-effects/bowel-dysfunction/
- **Details of Bowel Dysfunction**
  https://www.prostate.org.au/awareness/further-detailed-information/understanding-prostate-cancer-treatments-and-side-effects/understanding-bowel-disturbance/managing-bowel-issues-after-prostate-cancer-diagnosis
- **Surgery and Bowel Movement**
  https://www.google.com/search?q=prostate+cancer+surgery+and+bowel&ie=UTF-8&oe=UTF-8&hl=en-us&client=safari

Bladder (Peeing) Dysfunction

According to the medical community, it is *normal to* have difficulty peeing and holding back urine after catheter removal. This is called urinary incontinence. Most patients use pads or adult diapers to control leaking urine, sometimes for up to one year. This medical community definition simplifies the actual issues and challenges the patient faces in managing the ability to pee post prostate cancer treatment(s). To a survivor, the lack of control is anything but *normal*!

Why? The prostate gland is in close proximity to multiple other organs (bladder, urinary gland, bowel tracks, localized nerves, and muscles), so the trauma of both the treatment and catheter tube will *absolutely* result in some form of peeing dysfunction. The level of dysfunction will vary greatly from one patient to another ranging from no control to limited control.

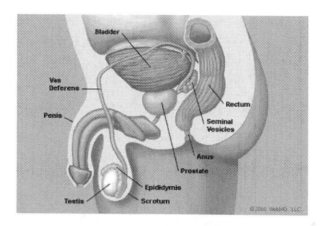

There is no way a patient will not be facing some level of peeing dysfunction. Some men do not have significant or long-term dysfunction. Others will experience dysfunction for at least one year or more, One fellow prostate survivor indicated no significant or long-term issues, but he did need to learn to pee again. The peeing issues and challenges a patient will face will be nothing but *abnormal!*

The level of dysfunction will vary greatly from one patient to another, and may include:

1. No ability to urinate standing up or sitting;
2. Dribbling of urine only into diapers;
3. Ablility to urinate lying on back or sideways into a urine bottle;
4. Ability to produce short streams or squirts of urine on cue; and/or
5. Passing of gas (farting) while peeing.

When will incontinence end?

The ability to control peeing will be improving when you are able to dribbling, squirt, or produce a short or long stream on cue. The medical community indicates there is a three-phase sequence for incontinence ending

1. After lying down;
2. After sitting; and
3. After walking.

Resources: Bladder/Peeing

- **Surgery and Bladder**
  https://www.webmd.com/urinary-incontinence-oab/mens-guide/urinary-incontinence explains how the bladder works and how surgery impacts it.
- **Continence and Prostate**
  https://www.continence.org.nz/pages/Continence-and-Prostate/37/ provides a definition of Kegel exercises and information.
- **Incontinence after Catheter Removal**
  https://www.cancerresearchuk.org/about-cancer/cancer-chat/thread/incontinence-immediately-after-catheter-removal
- **Were You Prepared For Incontinence?**
  http://paact.help/were-you-prepared-for-incontinence-after-prostate-cancer-treatment-by-sarah-woodward-bioderm-inc-2013/
- **What Are Actual Rates of Incontinence? (Lies, damn lies!)**

http://www.smsna.org/sandiego2016/presentations/006.pdf

- **Urinary Problem Treatment: Sling**
https://prostatecanceruk.org/prostate-information/living-with-prostate-cancer/urinary-problems
- **Peeing Positions**
https://www.adisc.org/forum/threads/peeing-position-challenge.55866/
- **Peeing: How to Pee Lying Down**
https://www.adisc.org/forum/threads/how-to-pee-while-laying-down.87304/
- **A Patient's Story: Overcoming Incontinence**
https://www.health.harvard.edu/blog/a-patients-story-overcoming-incontinence-2009031125

- Additional PC information provided in Chapter 20: PC Resources.

Sexual Dysfunction

As for sex and intimacy, many men worry about having sexual dysfunction and inability to have an erection. The inability to have an erection and perform sexually is one of the most complex elements of the recovery process for most men. It not only impacts the patient in the most private arena of his personal life, it also deeply affects his relationship with another person. The physiology and psychology of the sex drive is already complicated enough without adding dysfunction into the mix.

The literature covering the issue of sexual dysfunction presents a realistic picture of the multiple issues involved. The level of dysfunction and recovery will vary greatly from one man to another, from full functionality to non-functionality. Dysfunction may include the following.

- Inability to have children
- No or minimal erection to full erection
- No ejaculation
- Impotence (the inability to achieve or maintain an erection) is a major side effect of most treatments for advanced prostate cancer. Among men who have both their testicles removed by a surgery known as orchiectomy, about 90 percent will experience impotence. Drugs to reduce testosterone levels, called androgen deprivation therapy or ADT, also cause impotence in most men. If this therapy is discontinued, many but not all men can regain erections over time with no assistance. Treatments to improve erections include medicines taken orally or injected into the penis, vacuum erection devices, and penile implants. Discuss these options with your doctor including their likelihood of success and patient satisfaction before you have treatment that may result in impotence.

The what, when, where, and how for recovery is largely unpredictable; you will need to be patient. Contact your medical community (doctor, hospital, PC organizations) where support, information, resources, and consultations are available to help you make decisions and process any sexual dysfunction. You may find the podcast *Mr. 80 Percent* helpful, as it covers sexual dysfunction issues.

Resources: Sexual Dysfunction

Sex Articles

- **Sexual Dysfunction Following Prostate Surgery**
  https://www.fredhutch.org/en/news/releases/2000/01/
  JAMAprostatectomy.html
- **Side Effects of Incontinence on Sex**
  https://www.google.com/search?q=prostate+cancer+
  surgery+and+sexuality&ie=UTF-8&oe=UTF-
  8&hl=en-us&client=safari
- **Viagra for Impotence Following Prostate Surgery**
  https://www.webmd.com/erectile-dysfunction/news/
  19991130/viagra-useful-impotence-following-
  prostate-surgery
- **Quality Outline Sex Overview**
  https://www.hopkinsmedicine.org/brady-urology-
  institute/patient-information/_docs/dr.handischarge_
  instructions.pdf

Sex Podcasts

- **Sex After Prostate Cancer**
  https://zerocancer.org
- ***Mr. 80 Percent***
  https://www.wbur.org/onpoint/2020/09/25/prostate-
  cancer-an-all-too-common-disease-thats-rarely-
  talked-about

- Additional PC information provided in Chapter 20:
  PC Resources.

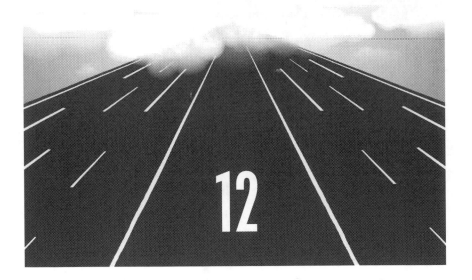

STRESS: PSYCHOLOGY OF CANCER

- Are you worried that prostate cancer will kill you?
- Are you having a hard time coming to grips with a prostate cancer diagnosis?
- Prostate cancer treatment(s) will be the start of a highly stressful life situation. Your subconscious stress may be creating vision, muscle tightness, headaches…without you even realizing it is happening.

Overview

Prostate cancer will be mentally and physically taxing on both the patient and caregiver.

The following information and links provide a deep dive into the mental and emotional aspects of recovery. Understanding the psychological impacts of cancer will enable you to better navigate the stress and trauma associated with being diagnosed with cancer. Prostate cancer survivors and medical professionals share a wide variety of insights to help the patient and caregiver deal with conscious and subconscious stress.

Is your jaw aching? Are your shoulders tight? How are you sleeping?

Though a patient's immediate response to these questions may be "I'm doing fine," the body may have a different answer. The body has a defense mechanism at work constantly to protect us, even when we are unaware of the tension building up within us. The actual and subconscious stress from having cancer and the trauma caused by the treatment can result in a wide variety of stress symptoms. The patient and caregiver need to monitor the body's reactions to alleviate any negative reactions.

Insights and Tips

Ten weeks after my surgery, I thought I was feeling great. I was getting back to my old routine, including working around the house and regular rounds of golf...then *bam*! All of a sudden, my eyes wouldn't focus, my equilibrium was way off, and my neck and shoulders muscles were extremely tight. I was shocked and extremely upset. As a male, reaching out to the doctor to talk about it didn't seem "manly." But my equilibrium was so off, I contacted my optometrist and other doctors, explaining that I was experiencing a focus and equilibrium problem, which felt like a combination of migraine and vertigo. Before my appointments, I tried to continue my normal routine, but it quickly became clear that this wasn't a good idea.

When I finally met with the doctors, no one could give me an answer as to why this was happening. On the upside, they found no structural damage to the eyes and ruled out any new illness or disease. However, I was left to my own devices. Of course, I jumped onto the internet to get some answers, and after hours of research I concluded that stress was the culprit. Through a combination of ice, heat, meditation, covering my eyes, exercising, stretching, using my rowing machine, and walking, I worked to alleviate the negative reaction.

Seven days later, my eyesight was better. I can't express enough the importance of being aware of any stress you might be harboring, and figuring out ways to proactively resolve it. This is definitely easier said than done. Just because the doctor turns you loose doesn't mean you are ready to jump back into your normal activities, full steam ahead. Do all you can to recognize and mitigate stress throughout your recovery process.

Resources: Stress

- **How To Handle Relapse of Cancer**
  https://www.health.harvard.edu/blog/how-to-handle-a-relapse-after-treatment-for-prostate-cancer-2009031122
- **Men and Prostate Cancer: The Emotional Aspect**
  https://www.cityofhope.org/prostate-emotional-issues
  The City of Hope blog provides patients a succinct overview of the adverse effects of prostate cancer and

treatment, as well as avenues available to address these impacts.

- **Emotional and Psychological Distress Associated With PC**
  https://www.ascopost.com/issues/september-25-2017/emotional-and-psychological-distress-associated-with-prostate-cancer/ is a brief article from ASCO (American Society of Clinical Oncology) with information on prostate cancer treatment, stress, and coping strategies.

- **Psychological Aspects of Prostate Cancer: A Clinical Review**
  https://www.nature.com/articles/pcan201166

- **Subtle Symptoms of Chronic Stress**
  https://www.activebeat.com/diet-nutrition/7-subtle-chronic-stress-symptoms/

- **10 Effects of Chronic Stress**
  https://www.activebeat.com/your-health/10-effects-of-chronic-stress-on-your-health/

Resources: Holistic Therapy Treatments

- **Holistic Therapies and Practices That Help With Anxiety and Depression**
  https://www.takingcharge.csh.umn.edu/what-holistic-therapies-and-practices-help-anxiety-and-depression
  From the University of Minnesota, Earl E. Bakken Center for Spirituality and Healing, this article gives a succinct overview of:

- Mind-body practices;
- Mindfulness and yoga;
- Nutritional supplements;
- Nature-based therapies;
- Animal-assisted and pet therapies;
- Music therapy;
- Traditional Chinese medicine; and
- Naturopathic medicine.

- **Holistic Stress Management for Mind, Body, and Spirit**
  https://www.holistic-mindbody-healing.com/holistic-stress-management.html

- **Holistic Treatment for Chronic Stress**
  https://ndnr.com/mindbody/jun-09-holistic-techniques-for-stress/

- **Meditation, Mindfulness, and Cancer: Can Meditation Help Cure Cancer?**
  https://www.headspace.com/blog/2017/04/16/meditation-and-cancer-patients/

- **Meditation as An Alternative Therapy**
  https://www.verywellhealth.com/meditation-for-people-with-cancer-2248959

- **Meditation for Neck and Shoulder Pain**
  https://www.youtube.com/watch?v=MypjOs5ZC8c
  This YouTube guide provides a short, simple, and gentle yoga practice that can help relieve neck and shoulder stiffness.

- **Guided Meditations for Cancer Patients (Excellent Viewpoints)**
  https://www.healthjourneys.com/guided-meditation-for-cancer-patients

- **Guided Meditation Apps**
  https://www.doyogawithme.com/content/guided-meditations-help-fight-cancer
- **Anxiety Relaxation Scripts**
  https://www.innerhealthstudio.com/anxiety-relief-scripts.html

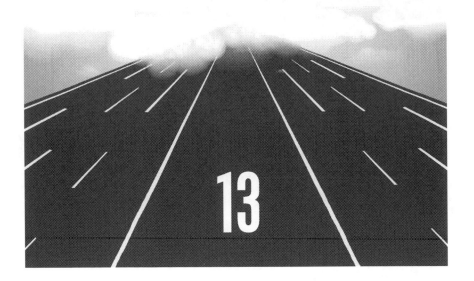

WALKING AND ACTIVITY OVERVIEW

- How much walking is enough for recovery? How far? How fast?

Overview

Walking and exercise are considered keys to healing. The body experiences a wide range of trauma and dysfunction after cancer treatments. Following treatment, your medical team will instruct you to walk early and often, up to five to six times per day. This direction is designed to get you up, out of bed, and moving, so your key body functions will return to normal as quickly as possible. To create a strong foundation for your walking practice, you may want to work with your medical team to formulate a plan of action. Studies show that patients who set goals, outline a plan, and draft a contingency list summarizing how they will overcome challenges and setbacks in getting back on their feet after surgery, have drastically better post-op outcomes.

Insights and Tips

According to a 2014 study, exercise may increase your chances of long-term prostate cancer survival.[1] Whether it is a few steps taken inside the house or a sixty-minute walk outside, it all counts. The duration of each outing will vary based on where you are in your healing process.

- **Monitor your energy:** The duration and intensity of your walks should be based on how you feel and your level of energy at the beginning of each session. Don't overdo it.
- **Move whenever you can:** Walking inside or outside, it all counts.
- **Change it up:** Add variety to your routine. Each walking session doesn't need to be the same—just get your walks in throughout the day.
- **Incremental progress is key:** The focus should be on making consistent progress, not distance or speed. Success is all about progressively building up your strength and stamina.
- **Set reminders:** Consider setting an alarm to ring every hour and a half to remind yourself to get your walk in.

Start by counting steps, then move to counting minutes, and build your practice by incorporating other activities (yard work, golf, hunting, running, biking, and so on) as your body and the doctor will allow. Each day, add more steps or time to what you had done the previous day. *Slow and steady*

---

[1] Stephanie E. Bonn, et al., "Physical activity and survival among men diagnosed with prostate cancer," *Cancer Epidemiology, Biomarkers & Prevention* 24, no. 1 (January 1, 2015): 57–64, https://doi.org/10.1158/1055-9965.EPI-14-0707.

progress is the key. Keep a log of your daily walking with the Recovery Walking Tracker, available as a PDF download at https://www.prostateroadmap.com/prostate-recovery-walking-exercise-info.

While recovery can feel painfully slow and tedious at times, tracking your activity can help you see tangible progress over time. Celebrate the little wins, from week to week, and one month to the next. During your first week of recovery, the bulk of your walking may be indoors, with only 150 to 500 steps taken per session. The following week, when the catheter has been removed, you might do a combination of indoor and outdoor walks, with between 500 and 1000 steps per session. By the third week, you might do a combination of indoor and outdoor walks and use either steps or minutes as your tracking metric.

Resources: Walking

- **Value of Walking Early**
  https://www.uwhealth.org/healthfacts/surgery/6711.html
- **Importance of Exercise**
  https://www.virginiamason.org/exercise-after-prostate-removal
- **Walking After Surgery Is Important**
  https://www.uwhealth.org/healthfacts/surgery/6711.html
- **Tracking Your Walking**
  https://www.verywellfit.com/tracking-your-walks-3432825

- **Benefits of Stretching**
  https://healthprep.com/articles/living-healthy/
  health-benefits-of-stretching/4/?utm_source=google
- **Diet and Prostate Cancer**
  https://www.healthline.com/health/prostate-cancer/
  prostate-cancer-and-diet

Walking Tracker Worksheet

Tracking Metrics
Steps: 100–250, 250–500, 500–1000, 1000–2000
Minutes: 3–5, 5–10, 10–15, 15–20, 20–30, 30–45,
45–60, 60+

Tracker Codes
Pace Level: Slow, Medium, Brisk
Tracking Type: S = Steps; M = Minutes
Location: H =House; Y = Outside
Energy Level: Low, Medium, High

Example 1: (S 60S H L) slow pace, 60 steps, house,
low energy

Example 2: (M 6M Y M) medium pace,6 Min,
Outside, Medium Energy

DAY	WALK 1	WALK 2	WALK 3	WALK 4	WALK 5	WALK 6
1						
2						
3						
4						
5						
6						
7						
8						
9						
10						
11						
12						
13						
14						
15						
16						
17						
18						
19						
20						

PDF of the Recovery Walking Tracker is available for download at https://www.prostateroadmap.com/prostate-recovery-walking-exercise-info.

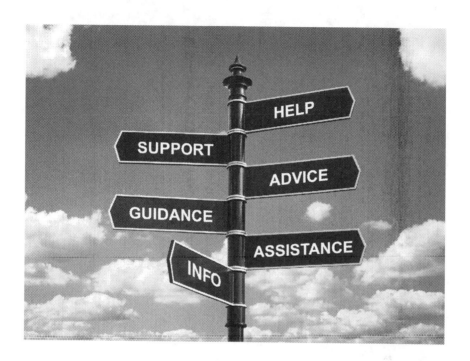

Note: Is there an easy way to connect to the URL links throughout the book? Yes, all URL'S provided can be accessed at https://www.prostateroadmap. com/ prostate-answers-articles-info. This will enable you to just click and read.

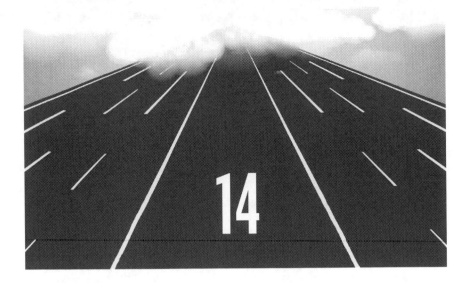

CAREGIVERS' SUPPORT RESOURCES

- How can you prepare for the journey ahead?
- What do you need to know to be part of the team!
- Survivors and professionals provide resources and insights to help you make informed decisions and lower stress levels.

Overview

The caregiver role is essential. Cancer treatment and recovery can often be nearly as mentally and physically taxing for caregivers as it is for patients. The truth is that patients cannot do it alone. Your role as the caregiver is extremely valuable, whether or not it is immediately acknowledged and appreciated. The information and resources provided are meant to help the caregiver prepare and maintain a sense of dignity, control, and stability throughout the man's recovery process.

What to Expect

Review the catheter management and recovery issues, challenges, and side effect sections with the patient prior to or following the PC treatment. This will help you both be prepared for the recovery process ahead. It is important to be aware and listen as the patient moves through the different phases of recovery. This includes everything from managing stress (the patient's and your own), to recovery hygiene, to establishing a physical therapy and exercise routine.

Preparing the Living Space

When the patient returns home after treatment, the patient and caregiver will be making all the decisions. Setting up the patient's primary living space and obtaining the supplies needed for recovery prior to the patient returning home will lead to less stress for both the caregiver and patient.

Do not hesitate to contact your medical provider with questions

Home Recovery Needs Checklist

Many items can help make the patient's recovery easier and help with the healing process. A Home Recovery Needs Checklist can be found in PDF format at https://www.prostateroadmap.com/prostate-homerecovery-needs-list.

Home Recovery Needs Store

If you are missing any of the items on the checklist from your medicine cabinet, go to the Home Recovery Needs Store https://www.prostateroadmap.com/prostate-home-recovery-needs-store). While most items can be purchased at your local pharmacy or supermarket, the Home Recovery Needs Store provides a wide range of competitively priced recovery aids all in one place, saving you time, energy, and money. Check everything off your list and order the supplies you need.

The purchased items will be shipped for free. The recovery supplies are only available in the United States.

Resources: Caregiver Articles

- **Your Cancer Game Plan**
  http://www.yourcancergameplan.com/people-living-with-cancer?
- **Common Complications and Concerns After Surgery**
  https://www.verywellhealth.com/common-problems-after-surgery-3156807. VeryWellHealth highlights potential problems to be on the lookout for post-treatment.
- **Understanding the Cancer Experience When You're a Caregiver**
  https://www.cancer.org/treatment/caregivers/what-a-caregiver-does/treatment-timeline.html. One of the first steps after being told someone you love has cancer will be learning about his diagnosis. This Cancer.org resource helps you understand the disease process and provides guidance on the first questions

that you and the patient should be asking the doctor and/or the cancer care team.

- **Making Health Decisions as a Cancer Caregiver** https://www.cancer.org/treatment/caregivers/ what-a-caregiver-does/making-decisions.html. This Cancer.org resource helps loved ones and caregivers navigate the sometimes challenging decision making landscape.

- **Urinary Catheter Care for Caregivers** https://elizz.com/caregiver-resources/urinary-catheter-care-for-caregivers/. For caregivers supporting a patient with a urinary catheter, this article provides catheter care tips that will help reduce the risk of problems and highlight concerns that may need assessment by the patient's health care provider.

- **Caring for someone with incontinence** https://www.continence.org.au/incontinence/carers. Many family members and friends find caring for a person with incontinence to be one of the most difficult aspects of caregiving. Incontinence can be unpredictable, add dramatically to your workload, and be very costly. Many caregivers report feeling angry, frustrated, lonely, and not able to cope as they try to manage alone. The Continence Foundation of Australia website offers practical information to assist you in your care.

- **Top 10 Items You Should Have at Home After a Surgery** https://www.verywellhealth.com/things-to-have-at-home-after-your-surgery-3156905

- **Getting your home ready after the hospital** https://medlineplus.gov/ency/patientinstructions/000432.htm. Getting your home ready after you have been in the hospital often requires much preparation. This article from Medline provides ideas on how patients can remain safe and healthy in their homes after treatment.

- **Follow-Up Care for Prostate Cancer:** https://www.cancer.net/cancer-types/prostate-cancer/follow-care. To help doctors provide their patients with the highest quality care, the American Society of Clinical Oncology (ASCO) issued an endorsement of a guideline developed in 2014 by the American Cancer Society. This guideline provides recommendations for follow-up care for men who have received treatment for prostate cancer.
- **Podcast: Patients and Family Support**
  https://podcast.mskcc.org/

- Additional PC information provided in Chapter 20: PC Resources.

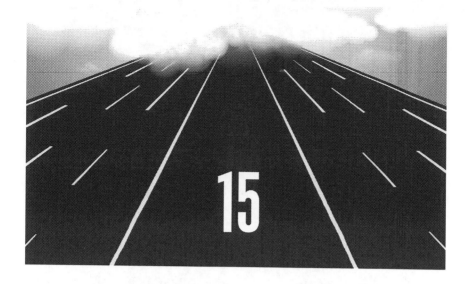

CHECKLIST FOR HOME RECOVERY NEEDS

■ What items will you need at home after PC treatment?

Home Recovery Needs Checklist

I. Bedroom and Bathroom

____ Absorbent floor pads*

____ Paper towels

____ Plastic bags

____ Diapers/guards*

____ Antibacterial soap*

____ Waste basket

____ Toilet bowl cleaner and brush

____ Protective bed pad*

____ Rags and old towels

____ Disinfectant spray

____ Sanitary wipes*

____ Kleenex

II. Personal Aids

____ Toothbrush and toothpaste

____ Chap Stick

____ Deodorant

____ Fan

____ Extra pillow

____ Eye drops

____ Hand lotion

____ Hair dryer

____ Entertainment: books, TV

____ Urine bottle*

____ Donut hole pillow*

____ Sleeping knee pad*

____ Jock strap*

____ Digital thermometer*

____ Pen, pencil, and paper

____ Clipboard or three-ring binder

____ Loose clothes for walking

____ Mouthwash

____ Water bottle

____ Absorbent guards/diapers*

____ Sleeping wedge pillow*

____ Brief underwear*

____ Body powder*

III. Healing Aids

____ Ice packs*

____ Acetaminophen

____ Antibiotic ointment

____ Salve ointment

____ Stool softener pills

____ Prune juice

____ Hemorrhoid ointment

____ Athlete's foot cream (Clotrimazole)

IV. Support Aids

____ Bedside table/stand

____ Catheter tube anchor

____ Computer table stand

____ ACE bandage*

____ Digital alarm clock*

____ Walking tracker

____ Walking watch*

____ Velcro straps*

____ Catheter strap*

A PDF of the Recovery Checklist is available for download at https://www.prostateroadmap.com/_files/ugd/71073b_1339dfd790ad4f0088aa1f61de0cb27a.pdf.

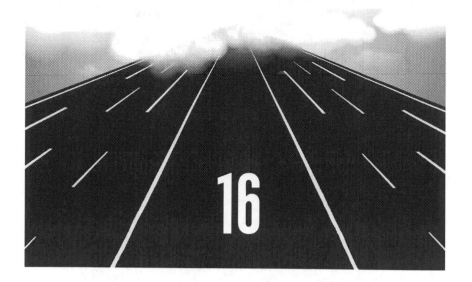

HOME RECOVERY NEEDS CHECKLIST DETAILS

- What, where, and why for checklist.

Overview

The details below provide insights and tips regarding the needed recovery supplies.

Hygiene

— **Rags and Towels:** Leaking, dribbling, and squirting urine necessitate having multiple rags or towels available throughout your living space.

— **Showers:**

■ **With catheter**: Identify where to hang the bag prior to treatment. The bag itself has a clothes hanger style hook, so you may be able to hang it on the shower door, a towel rack, or the shower fixture itself. Showering with a catheter is not overly complicated; just make sure the hose doesn't get pulled out!

- ■ **Post-Catheter:** Due to leakage when wearing a diaper or guard, it is critical to keep your body clean. An easy way to do a quick clean without taking a full shower is to stand with one foot in the shower and wash the area(s) that need to be cleaned. You may find it necessary to take multiple showers per day for the first few weeks.

Personal Aids

- — **Absorbent Guards Option 1:** These are essential for protection after the catheter is removed. Absorbent guards will handle most of the leakage. You will need brief underwear to hold it in place. They are available at your local drug/grocery stores.
- — **Adult Diapers Option 2:** You may only need to rely on diapers for the first few days after the catheter is removed, so purchase a smaller amount initially. Diapers can be purchased at your local drug/grocery stores. The diapers will create a great deal of heat.
- — **Urine Bottle:** Having a urine bottle on hand can be crucial until normal bladder control returns. Whether you pee standing up, lying on your side on the bed, in a chair, or on your back, a clean urine bottle will help get you through the ordeal of being unable to hold and/ or control urine. The urine bottles are not typically

available at your local drugstore but may be found at local medical supply companies or ordered online at www.prostateroadmap.com.

— **Jock Strap:** A jock strap is an effective alternative to wearing brief underwear to hold absorbent guards in place. It can also be helpful when moving around for prolonged periods, exercising, or participating in sport activities. Wearing a jock strap to support the guard with boxer shorts over them will not generate as much heat as the briefs. While not typically available at retail stores, jock straps can be found online at www.prostateroadmap.com.

Healing Items

— **Ice Packs:** Useful to reduce swelling and speed up healing:
  - On perineum area between legs
  - On both sides of scrotum
  - On lower abdomen (including stitches)

  Wrap ice packs in an old tee shirt or cloth rag to protect your skin from frostbite. Store two sets of ice packs in freezer bags, with two packs in each freezer bag. Limit icing to ten to fifteen minutes three times per day.

— **Antibiotic ointment (with catheter):** Bacitracin, A&D ointment, and others

— **Antibiotic ointment (post catheter):** Athlete's foot cream with
  Clotrimazole, Bacitracin, A&D Ointment. Athlete's foot cream can be a lifesaver if you get a yeast infection

from wearing the diapers/guards. Apply as directed, liberally and often, to minimize rashes and protect against infection. The yeast infection can have a fishy odor. Even if the penis looks healed, that doesn't mean the infection is gone. As long as there is odor, continue applying the athlete's foot ointment until the odor is gone.

Support Aids

— **Catheter Bedside Set-up** (hose *must* be below bag). Setting-up the tube at the bedside can be done as follows.
  ▪ Have Velcro strips available.
  ▪ Use an anchor item: use a folding chair, short stool, table, or ladder.
  ▪ Connect the tube to the anchor items with the Velcro strips.
  ▪ Place the anchor at a distance that will allow enough leeway between bed and catheter bag.
  Using the anchor provides safety as it will stabilize the tubing. Do not allow the bag to touch the ground or lay on the floor. Handing the bag inside a waste basket can protect against accidental spills. The hose itself can lay on the floor.
— **Hanging a Catheter Bag:** The catheter bag has a built-in hook. Take time to review possible hanging locations:
  ▪ Shower
  ▪ Bedside

- Kitchen
- Near Toilet
- Sitting Areas

— **Bedside Stand:** Place a designated stand next to the bed where you can easily place and reach the urine bottle, light switch, alarm, tissues, reading material, and other items. This can be any folding chair, low table, footstool, or other stand that you have available.

— **Cloth Rag/Coaster:** Place under bottle.

General Tips

— **Kegel/Pelvic Floor Exercise:** It is vital to prepare your body for bladder issues after treatment. Make sure to establish a daily routine and start Kegel exercises *prior* to surgery. There are many online resources where you can teach yourself, or ask your doctor for a physical therapy pelvic floor referral.

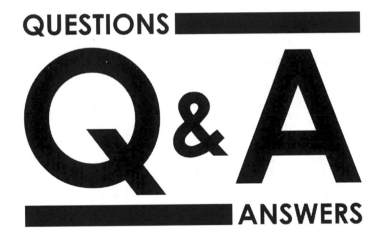

Paul Surface

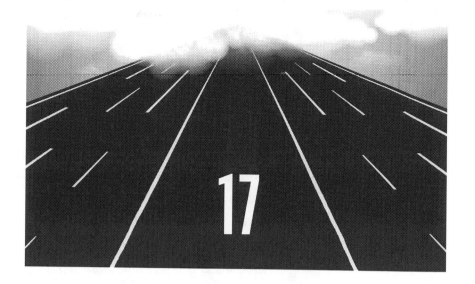

PROSTATE CANCER
QUESTIONS AND ANSWERS

- Do you have questions about PC issues that may be embarrassing?
- Do you have questions that weren't adequately addressed by your doctor and/or are particularly sensitive?
- This chapter covers everything from urinary and sexual dysfunction, to constipation, hygiene, and life during and after wearing a catheter. Examples include the challenges of body dysfunction (peeing, sexual issues, constipation), hygiene, and wearing a catheter.

Overview

The prostate cancer recovery journey can seem like a maze, full of twists, turns, and dead ends. Patients receive varying degrees of information from their treatment providers regarding what to expect after treatment and how to prepare for recovery. The answers found in the sampling of questions and answers are from fellow prostate cancer survivors, who share experiences from their own recovery journeys. The sampling is compiled to provide patients and caregivers with answers as they navigate and manage the PC issues and challenges they face.

The questions and answers provided in the book are a sampling of questions and answers that have been resourced and compiled. Additional questions and answers can be found at https://www.prostateroadmap.com/prostate-qna-recovery-answers-info.

A: Diagnosis and Tests

Q. How long will I live?
A. Everyone is different. No two patients are entirely alike, as treatment and responses to treatment can vary greatly. Your personal recovery experience will be impacted by treatment choice, age, any additional health factors, the treatment side effects, and your body's response to treatment.

Q. What should I know (or should have known) prior to treatment?
A. There are a wide variety of issues and challenges a patient will face after treatment. Becoming knowledgeable about the following would be a good place to start.

- Learn about the range of items you might need during recovery and how to prepare your home by reviewing the Recovery Checklist Section.
- Start Kegel exercises as soon as you are aware your selected treatment will require the support of a catheter during your recovery.

- Get your affairs in order ahead of time. Read the Cancer Realities page to gain insight into a wider range of considerations you'll need to contend with during your cancer journey.
- If your recovery will include a catheter:
  - Become familiar with the different ways to stabilize the unit.
  - Learn how to prepare your bedroom for sleeping with a catheter.
  - Learn how to secure the unit for walking.
- After the catheter is removed:
  - Be aware of the voiding process.
  - Be prepared to experiment with different peeing positions throughout recovery.
  - Learn about potential side effects and how to mitigate them.
- Review our walking and exercise overview and familiarize yourself with how to track your progress.

B: Deciding on a Treatment Option

Q. Which PC treatment should I choose?

A. Talk about stress! It all starts with doing your research by learning all the pros and cons of each treatment option. My choice was easy, due to my cancer being deemed aggressive. My doctor told me I owed it to myself to get a second opinion. Typically, a doctor will recommend the treatment that is his or her specialty, so it is important to get opinions from doctors of different specialties. It all comes down to doing your research and choosing the option and medical team that seems most comfortable for you. The bottom line is to be you own advocate. Fortunately, due to the advancements of cancer medicine, multiple cancer treatment options allow millions of people to live long, productive lives after treatment.

C: Challenges: Urinary and Bowel Issues

Q. What should my expectation be regarding peeing once the catheter is removed?
A. Some individuals have limited interruption and control of their bladder function, while others have to teach themselves to pee again normally.

Q. Why is urination such a problem after catheter removal?
A. It is a combination of proximity, stitches and swelling, nerve damage, removal of a body part, removal of nerves, and the disturbance of the body's basic functions as a result of treatments that play a part in the disruption of bladder control. What happens? All the reading material indicates it takes time for the brain to be in communication with your bladder and signal that it is time to pee. (You will not find any of these descriptions and definitions in a textbook or dictionary.)

Q. **Is it bad that I can only pee into a urine bottle while lying on my side and not while standing up?**
A. No, it all counts.

Q. Do I need a urine bottle?
A. Yes, after the catheter has been removed.

Q. Will leakage ever stop?

A. For many patients, the answer is yes. Then there those of us who will manage the leakage forever. Even if you start with the worst possible bladder dysfunction, the body does heal and you will regain bladder control. At some point, you will be excited to be able to stand or walk without dribbles and be able to pee again normally. If after one year, you're still experiencing life-impacting dysfunction, you can talk to your doctor about the sling surgical option.

Q. Is it normal to squirt every time I get out of a chair or bed? Or when leaning over or picking up something heavy?

A. Yes, it is one of those normal abnormals. It is amazing how much the lower core is in play when you make even the slightest movement. Doing Kegel exercises will strengthen these muscles. You may want to continue doing the exercises, even after you have regained control over your peeing.

Q. Is it normal to fart while peeing? I did not have that issue before the surgery.

A. Yes, the farting while peeing is just one additional possible side effect. You may be surprised to learn that many men experience this issue even if they never had surgery!

Q. Is it normal for my poop to be hard as a rock?

A. My first poop was hard as a rock due to the anesthesia, so easy does it. Use a stool softener, plus have hemorrhoid medicine available.

D. Diaper Rash or Yeast Infection

Q. Is it possible I have diaper rash or a yeast infection?
A. Yes, both are possible side effects of having to wear a diaper or guard. Diapers create a moist, humid atmosphere, and wearing a urine-soiled diaper a little too long is a perfect recipe for a fungal infection.

It took three days of experimentation for me to clear up my yeast infection. For the first two days, I tried a combination of ointments: A&D antibiotic cream and zinc oxide with some baby powder thrown into the mix. Nope, that didn't work, so I moved on to a couple of home remedies. First, I applied diluted hydrogen peroxide, then apple cider vinegar dabbed onto the scrotum. Not only did they not work, the scrotum stung so bad I decided there was no way in hell I was going to go through that pain for up to two weeks in hopes that it would work.

I immediately drove to the closest drugstore, searched in the yeast infection section, but found nothing for men and asked the pharmacist for help. I was directed to the athlete's foot section. I was hesitant because there were no big letters stating this athlete's foot medicine product works on a man's yeast infection. It just said athlete's foot cream with clotrimizole. Well, there was no way I was going back to the vinegar, so I gave the cream a try. Within fifteen hours, the area didn't look like hamburger and the redness was gone. I continued to use the ointment for one week and never had to confront this scary issue again.

E: Pain

Q. What types of pain should I expect?

A. Surprisingly, I experienced only minor pain as a result of my prostate cancer treatment. The painkillers from surgery will remain in your system for a few days, so don't get too exuberant and walk too much or too fast too soon. Otherwise, you will pay the next day, as I did. Types of pain you may experience include the following.

- **Stomach:** The stomach surgery area will remain bloated and feel tight from wrestling with the robotic machinery. For me, it was somewhat uncomfortable and my movement was limited for a week or so, but I had no major pain.
- **Stitches:** The stitches caused no pain sensation. They were extremely hot during the first week, so I used ice packs to help them heal. Instructions say to keep them dry and not put any ointment on them. I missed those instructions the first few weeks, but no harm no foul.
- **Penis:** The inserted catheter will generate pain on your penis tip when not secured properly. Sitting with the catheter in place will be at a minimum uncomfortable, due to the way the catheter tube runs under your body. When sitting, the tube compresses against the area between your legs called the perineum and it was too painful for me to sit. In fact, I had residual pain and couldn't sit comfortably for four weeks after surgery, which I initially blamed on the catheter tube. Once my nerve endings started to regenerate, I realized the pain was due to a combination of the catheter tube and removal of the prostate.

- **Nerve regeneration:** That final pain was the regeneration of the nerve endings about three and a half week after surgery. Up to that point, there had been no pain sensations or pain discomfort in the surgery areas or genitals. Once the nerves started the regeneration process, there was discomfort and intermittent sharp pains. Nothing was major or of long duration, but the area was tender.

Q. Why would I feel sharp pains in the lower abdominal area after three weeks when there was no pain earlier?
A. You may experience sharp pains during your recovery as the nerves impacted during treatment begin to regenerate

F: Home Recovery Needs Preparation: Diapers or Pads?

Q. How do I know what to buy, in what size, and how many before treatments?
A. I found guards to be better for daytime, while diapers initially were better for me at night. I stopped using diapers after three weeks, however, because they were too hot. I am not sure you even need the diapers, because it is leakage you are dealing with.

G: Walking and Exercise

Q. How many steps or minutes am I expected to walk during my five to six walks per day?
A. Walking is considered to be one of the most important components of recovery. Whether it is a short or long walk

outside or steps taken inside, it all counts. The amount is totally dependent on where you are in your healing process. Check out the Walking and Exercise section for more insight and resources.

Q. How soon after PC treatments should I start exercising?
A. Not too soon! You should strictly follow the doctor's recommendations and let your body heal on the inside. You don't want a setback. Just walk a lot!

H: General

Q. What are the risks of return of cancer?
A. Due to my aggressive cancer diagnosis, in 2019 my doctor told me he expects it to return. It has not returned yet. There are many statistics out there, but each man is different.

Q. Should I have my PSA tested?
A. Absolutely. Be your own advocate!

Q. What exactly is voiding?
A. The premise is that once the catheter is removed, you will need to make sure the bladder is working within the first six to twelve hours.

Q. What about Kegels?
A. The medical team did not bring up the need to do Kegels. I found out post-surgery. I wish I had been told.

I: When to Contact Your Medical Team/Call 911

Q. When should I contact my doctor after treatment?
A. Always seek the advice of your physician or other qualified health providers with any questions you may have regarding a medical condition.

- Additional PC Q@A can be found at prostateroadmap.com https://www.prostateroadmap.com/prostate-qn a-recovery-answers-info

Q. Do PSA scores fluctuate?

Q. Is a genetic test needed?

Q. What are the benefits of 3T MRI pre-biopsy? What can an MRI do?

Q. Should I wait and use active surveillance?

Q. Should I wait for treatment? The doctor is slow and in no hurry.

Q. Is incontinence a side effect of beam radiotherapy?

Q. Does the sphincter sling work?

Q. How much do PC treatments cost?

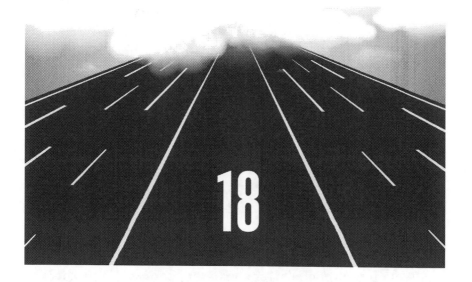

STORIES FROM FELLOW PC SURVIVORS

Fellow Prostate Cancer Survivors Sharing PC Journey Stories

Overview

I had no idea how my life would change after being diagnosed and choosing a prostatectomy. At this point, I am thankful to be alive, and that my cancer has not returned. I am making the most out of each day.

The survivor stories in the book are a sampling of questions and answers that have been resourced and compiled. Additional survivor stories can be found at https://www.prostateroadmap. com/prostate-recovery-challenges-tips

A: Diagnosis and Test Stories

Going through the diagnosis stage causes a great deal of stress.

- **Men's Stories of Prostate Cancer**
  https://www.cancer.org/latest-news/survivor-speaks-out-about-life-after-prostate-cancer.html
- **What happens after a prostate cancer diagnosis?**
  https://www.youtube.com/watch?v=nY0jYIj4r1I
- **Prostate Cancer Survivor Stories on YouTube**
  https://www.youtube.com/watch?v=faz_mtnG7lg

B. Survivor Treatment Stories

PC Treatment: Robotic Prostatectomy with Additional Hormone Treatment and Radiation

Survivor Story

Age at diagnosis: 77; Gleason score:8; Treatment type: Surgery, hormone, and radiation

I felt healthy, but then found out I had a raised PSA level. After months of antibiotics and being told it was nothing to worry about (a whole other topic) the doctor insisted on a biopsy. Prostate Cancer with a Gleason score of 8 was found. A radical prostatectomy was performed 6 weeks later.

At my first check up the PSA was 2.8, then microscopic amounts of cancer were found in my bladder and seminal vesicles. They began hormone therapy immediately and had radiation treatments 5 times a week for 8 week [*sic*] The catheter removed two weeks after surgery. I had already bought in a large supply of incontinence pads before the catheter was removed. The immediate effect of removal was that I couldn't pee at all and the hospital kept me waiting around (drinking coffee!) until I had actually managed to pass some water. After that, all my signals were mixed up and I had no idea whether I needed to go or not. That night I didn't get much sleep.

Eventually, my body reassociated the signals from the bladder with being full or empty and I was no longer running to the loo only to find there was nothing to pass. I was surprised (but in hindsight it was obvious) to find that I was passing a lot of blood clots with my urine. This continued for several months. Also my penis developed a massive bruise which wasn't painful. A colleague who'd been through this earlier warned me of this "Purple Ronnie" stage.

As instructed, I did the pelvic floor exercises several times every day. At this stage, I cut out all caffeine and went to de-caf tea and coffee. I stuck with this for about 8 months and then went back to the caffeinated versions. For the first month, although I could control when I wanted to go, any movement or cough or sneeze would release some urine into the pad. It was a little better lying down, but I still had to wear a pad 24/7 except in the shower. After about three months, the amount of leakage reduced considerably and I was able to stop using the full size pads and instead buy the much thinner Always Ultra pads instead. By the time six months was up, I was reliably 99.99% continent and leak free, so I stopped all pads; however I carried spare undies and a few spare pads in my briefcase. I only had one accident when I sneezed, but I was right outside a toilet and it wasn't a major incident.

After 8 months, I was confident enough to go on a day trip by train, wearing no pads, but still carrying some spares. I made sure that I emptied my bladder every 2-3 hours, just to avoid any build up of pressure. I still kept some precautions when I was sleeping, although I never had any accidents in bed. After a year, I gave up on all precautions and just went on as before. Since then I've had a couple of very minor accidents, losing no more than a drop of urine each time.

Over the years I've kept up with the Pelvic Floor exercises and the number of these small accidents has dropped to almost zero—in fact, I can't remember the last one. So, really it was a case of continual small improvements over a 6-8 month period. This, I think, is normal for most men. After surgery, a lot of healing has to take place, and I think that you shouldn't expect much improvement until you've stopped peeing out blood clots. I suggest you start now (before surgery) with the Pelvic Floor exercises, and continue with them for life.

One further hint. When you come home from surgery, you' [sic] be given an overnight catheter bag. PUT THIS IN A BUCKET. Almost everybody forgets to close up all the little valves at some time, and if you get it wrong you end up with a carpet full of **** as you sleep! It nearly happened to me, but fortunately my bag was in a bucket, and it didn't leak onto the floor. You should also expect to be very, very tired after surgery. For two weeks I would wake up… shower, and have breakfast then crawl back into bed until lunchtime. After lunch I could normally watch about an hour of TV, then crawl back into bed again and kip until about 6 pm. By 10 pm I was ready to go to bed and sleep right through to 8 am the next morning.

PC Survivor and Friend S.W.

PC Treatment: Robotic Prostatectomy

Survivor Story

22 years ago today, Aug 30, 1999, I had my prostatectomy surgery. I had just turned 48. I was diagnosed July 7th with PSA 4.4. It was detected by my family physician during a physical exam dre [sic] (my first in 7 years) who sent me to a urologist for biopsy. My first thoughts were that I would not grow old with my wife—we celebrate our 45th wedding anniversary in a couple months; I would not see my children grow up or see grandchildren—our children are grown and we have 6 wonderful grandchildren. My PSA has remained undetected requiring no further treatment.

However, several years after surgery, caused by numerous urinary tract infections, due to incontinence, I developed phimosis (tightening of the foreskin) requiring circumcision prior to having a sling installed, in 2012, to correct the incontinence. Within a year the sling broke requiring its removal. In 2014 I had surgery to install an AMS700CX penile implant—wish I had done it years before.

In 2015 I had an AMS800 Artificial Urinary Sphincter installed which has made the world of difference. I no longer have to go out loaded down with pads in case of not getting to a bathroom soon enough or checking a chair every time I got up hoping I hadn't left a wet spot.

At the time of my surgery, I joined a local prostate cancer support group and attended occasionally but I was 48 and they were a bunch of 'old guys' so I soon stopped attending—that was a mistake. A few years ago I went back to the group and have become involved in the leadership. I am not there so much for myself but for the 'new' guys who come with questions and fear. I encourage each of you if possible to connect with a local support group or start one. Our group is open to prostate cancer survivors and their families as well as anyone looking for information and support.

I joined this fb [sic] group a few years ago to learn from you in order to help others as there has been so much progress in the past 22 years. I have recommended this site to several people and see them encouraging others. We must each make our decisions as to the path we take and be comfortable with our decisions. I will soon be taking a break from this site but will check in from time to time. Keep up the good work and be patient with each other as we each face a different path. Each day I thank God for the time he has given me.

PC Survivor C. S.

PC Treatment: Hormonal Therapy

Survivor Story

Age at diagnosis: 64; current age: 69; treatment type: hormone therapy

The radiation may have been partially responsible for the surgery I had to have for a fistula from my colon to my bladder. I was hospitalized and was close to sepsis. I then had to have a portion of my colon removed. I had had diverticulitis before the radiation treatments and believe that the radiation was partially responsible.

Now two years after my hormone cancer treatment, I still have the side effects. Fatigue, I have to take Flomax, my penis seems smaller, I can have an erection but no sperm, my breasts are enlarged and I am now scheduled for a mammogram next week due to a small lump. Doesn't seem to end. My boobs have gotten so large due to the Hormone Therapy. Just found there is a way to undo that. Gynecomastia due to hormone therapy for advanced prostate cancer: a report of ten surgically treated cases and a review of treatment options.

PC Survivor and Friend W.W.

PC Treatment: Seeds

Survivor Story

Age at diagnosis: 69; treatment type: seed implant 4-9-19
PSA score pre-treatment: 2.1 to 4.2 to 5.2 over a one and a half year period
PSA score post-treatment: 1.02 to .27 over a one year period

Gleason score: 7

At any rate, what I was reading did not appear to be as applicable to my situation, though some of it does fit my circumstances, no doubt. With my treatment having been the seeds being implanted, I was able to fly from Ohio to FL the day after surgery and I never needed to use a catheter. In a nutshell, I seem to be getting along well, with a reasonably quick recovery and continued improvement to "the new normal.

PC Survivor and Friend R.L.

PC Treatment: Radiation, Lupron, Chemo

Survivor Story

Age: 59; treatment: radiation; Gleason score: 10
When I was diagnosed in October 2014, I had Stage 4 metastatic diagnosed with PC and given 6 months to live! Thankfully, that was 7 years ago! The cancer

had spread to my spine. Since it had already spread to my bones there was no need to remove the prostate, hence no surgery [*sic*] I had 10 rounds of radiation on my spine and left femur, followed by 6 rounds of chemo. I have been getting Lupron injections since I was diagnosed.

PC Survivor and Friend M.H.

Resources: Robotic Surgery and Radiotherapy

- **Robotic Surgery for Prostate Cancer** https://www.prostateprohelp.com/how-is-the-prostate-removed-in- robotic-surgery/
- **Surgery or Radiotherapy** https://www.youtube.com/watch?v=CAmOAeRQ0Ps

Resources: Hormone Therapy

- **Hormone Treatment Study** https://www.ncbi.nlm.nih.gov/pubmed/15510985/
- **Hormone and Chemotherapy** https://www.youtube.com/watch?v=Yq1Rr3R6UsM

Resource: Radiation

- **Radiation Therapy for PC on YouTube** https://www.youtube.com/watch?v=goyTxNuMCho

Resource: Immunotherapy

- **Prostate Cancer Immunotherapy Stories on YouTube**
  https://www.youtube.com/watch?v=uaa3RUVfTOg

The survivor stories in the book are a sampling of survivor stories that have been resourced and compiled.

Additional survivor stories can be found at https://www.prostateroadmap.com/prostate-recovery-challenges-tips

- **PC Treatments: Active Surveillance, Proton Beam Radiation**
- **PC Treatments: Lupron, Surgery**
- **PC Treatment: Cyberknife**
- **Issues, Challenges, and Side Effects Stories**
- **Pain in the Legs: Blood Clots After Surgery**
- **General Stories:**
- **Hiccups**
- **Undetectable**

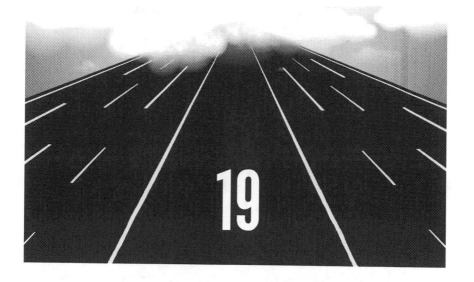

PC JOURNEY REALITIES
AND STATISTICS

Overview

A prostate cancer diagnosis is the start of a personal journey that will present emotional and psychological challenges for both patients and caregivers. Now that you have been told you have cancer, your view of life is changed forever. I immediately started to look at statistics on life expectancy after prostate cancer. Next, I turned to statistics on life expectancy for my age. The answer? The life expectancy for each was the same. Now that was a rude awakening!

Over the years, my expectation was that I would lead a long, long healthy life with no final number of years attached. It took a while to come to grips with the idea of having five, ten, fifteen, or twenty years to live. The challenge of dealing with the diagnosis of cancer puts us all in the position of facing our mortality, as uncomfortable as that may be. After wrestling with the idea for a few days, I decided to follow this mantra: "It's not how many days I have left, it's about what I make of the day…how I live and experience each day to make each day special."

Realities of Managing the Process: Each cancer patient ends up driving his or her own recovery. Each cancer has unique challenges for each patient; there is no single roadmap for treatment or management of the recovery process. So many decisions and actions will happen along the way. After the challenges of the initial diagnosis, treatment, and overall process, the cancer patient may still face the recurrence of cancer, followed by a second or third set of treatments for recovery and finally end-of-life decisions.

Realities of Treatment: The type of treatment used for cancer is dependent on the type of cancerous cell, stage of development, and age of the patient. Some patients will need to be treated aggressively, while others will be monitored by watchful waiting. It is daunting to realize that no matter what, cancer cannot be cured.

Realities of Variables: Each patient will have different experiences and reactions throughout his or her recovery journey. The experiences differ due to a multitude of variables: type of cancer cells, extent of surgery, patient's physical condition, type of treatment, the body's receptivity to surgery, the body's receptivity to healing, nerve regeneration, and so on. The list is as varied as each individual's DNA. The mystery of life becomes more profound the more I ponder having cancer.

Realities of Needing a Plan of Action: The patient and caregivers need to prepare a plan for as many contingencies as possible. Preparation before the cancer treatment can remove an additional layer of stress throughout your recovery.

Realities of Needing an Estate Plan: I finally took the time to put together a will, after knowing it was something I should do for years. I kept putting it off. What a weird feeling to complete a will, and being forced to come to grips with the reality of having cancer and my own mortality. This was just one more item on my action plan.

Realities Bottom Line: The PC journey process puts the patient and caregiver in new world of experiences that they will need to navigate and manage. Do the research to be able to make educated decisions, even if you will be at the steering wheel of a fixer upper heading down recovery lane. My best to you and your family throughout your PC journey.

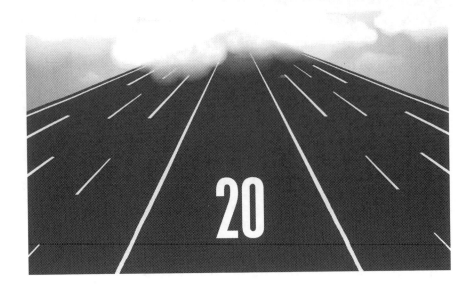

PC RESOURCES

- Are you looking for answers?

Overview

As a PC Advocate, I have continued my research to find resources that can be helpful for those diagnosed with Prostate Cancer. A PC diagnosis creates multiple questions. This chapter provides PC articles, resources, and reference URL links to support you and your caregivers as you make decisions throughout your PC journey.

Is there an easier way to connect to the URL links?

Instead of typing in each link, the compiled list provided below can also be found at https://www.prostateroadmap. com/prostate-answers-articles-info. This will enable you to just click and read.

Note: While every effort has been made to ensure the

accuracy and viability of the website addresses listed in this book, please know that some of these may have changed by the time of publication.

I. General:

FACEBOOK

- **Prostate Cancer Support Group**
  Ask a question, receive twenty to eighty replies!
- **Prostate Cancer Wives**
  Talk and support group (only women can join)
- **Prostate Cancer Non-Surgery Treatments Group**

WEBSITES

- **Prostate Cancer Roadmap**
  www.prostateroadmap.com
  This site has a library of links to cancer-related articles and non-surgery stories from survivors.
- **You Are Not Alone Support Group**
  www.yananow.com
  The You Are Not Alone website is a comprehensive, prostate-specific website. The site provides support to help you come to grips with a prostate cancer diagnosis. Articles include "Don't Panic," "What Did Other Men Do," and "Not Just a Man's Disease."
- **Prostate Cancer Foundation**
  www.pcf.org
  This website has information and a free brochure
- **American Cancer Society**
  www.cancer.org
  This site offers treatment and side effects information.

- **ZERO: The End of Prostate Cancer**
  www.zerocancer.org
  This site offers treatment and side effects information.
- **WebMD**
  www.webmd.com
  This site offers treatment and side effects information.
- **The Mayo Clinic**
  www.mayoclinic.org
  This site provides an overview of PC diagnosis and treatment.
- **Prostate Matters**
  www.prostatematters.co.uk
  This site has comprehensive PC information.
- **True North**
  www.truenorth.movember.com/en
- **Prostate Health Education Network**
  www.phenpsa.com
- **California Prostate Cancer Coalition**
  www.prostatecalif.org
- **Talk that Talk PC**
  https://www.talkthattalkpc.com/

ARTICLES
- **Internal Cancers**
  https://www.google.com/search?q=internal+cancers&ie=UTF-8&oe=UTF-8&hl=en-us&client=safari
- **Anesthesia: Frequently Asked Questions**
  http://www.gasdocs.com/faq.php
- **Does Cancer Return After Prostate Surgery?**
  https://www.google.com/search?q=does+prostate+cancer+return+at+the+site+of+the+prostate+if+the+prostate

+has+been+removed%3F&ie=UTF-8&oe=UTF-8&h
l=en-us&client=safari
- **Picture of Male Anatomy**
  https://www.emedicinehealth.com/image-gallery/
  prostate_picture/images.htm

II. Cancer Procedures and Treatments

- **Treatments and Statistics**
  https://www.urotoday.com/conference-highlights/
  astro-2021/133626-astro-2021-intermediate-risk-
  prostate-cancer-best-of-worlds-for-choices-worst-of-
  worlds-for-deciding.html?fbclid=IwAR0n
  NbrXAuO1uXS_OGTlSQKVMqNCQzaGtZF5Am
  MWiX5iEbx2VQppxTgD7fU
- **Prostate Cancer Stages and Grades for Diagnosis**
  https://www.cancer.net/cancer-types/prostate-
  cancer/stages-and-grades?fbclid=IwAR062pPrX
  XuXC-mSUcyq_GcBsPEVMgXF57dYcEzObQZ
  07ET2AAOpcz0tQso
- **Types of Treatment**
  - https://www.cancer.net/cancer-types/prostate-
    cancer/types-treatment
  - https://www.cancer.gov/types

Surgical Procedures
- **Prostate Cancer: Google Search**
  https://www.google.com/search?q=Prostate+cancer
  &ie=UTF-8&oe=UTF-8&hl=en-us&client=safari
- **Surgery for Prostate Cancer**

https://www.cancer.org/cancer/prostate-cancer/treating/surgery.html

- **Radical Prostatectomy: Q & A**
https://www.siumed.edu/surgery/urology/faqs-radical-prostatectomy.html
- **Surgical Side Effects**
https://zerocancer.org/learn/current-patients/side effects/

Radiation Therapy

- **Radiation Treatments**
https://www.cancercenter.com/treatment-options/radiation-therapy?invsrc=non_branded_paid_search_google&t_pur=prospecting&t_med=online&t_ch=paid_search&t_adg=59675573886&t_ctv=305585881401&t_mtp=b&t_pos=1t2&t_plc=kwd-298133032318&t_si=google&t_tac=none&t_con=non_brand&t_bud=corp&t_d=m&t_tar=non_targeted&t_aud=any&kxconfid=s8ymtai82&dskid={trackerid}&t_mod=cpc&t_cam=1604505103&t_trm=%2Bradiation%20%2Btreatment&t_src=g&dstrackerid=43700037991408012&gclsrc=aw.ds&&gclid=CjwKCAjwpuXpBRAAEiwAyRRPgZh5_iIDno7yZdatKxLU9uovoEnTE1I4oaKaWVE3IVKrvjI9Tw9F9RoCZQwQAvD_BwE
- **Considerations for Radiation Therapy**
https://www.cancerforums.net/threads/57224-Some-considerations-when-looking-a-radiation-therapy?highlight=PROSTATE

- **Radiation Side Effects**
  https://www.google.com/search?q=radiation+side+effects+prostatectomy&ie=UTF-8&oe=UTF-8&hl=en-us&client=safari

Hormone Therapy
- **Hormone Therapy for Prostate Cancer**
  https://www.cancer.org/cancer/prostate-cancer/treating/hormone-therapy.html
- **Types of Hormone Therapy**
  https://www.cancer.org/cancer/prostate-cancer/treating/hormone-therapy.html
- **Side Effects of Prostate Hormone Therapy**
  https://www.google.com/search?q=side+effects+of+hormone+therapy+for+prostate+cancer&ie=UTF-8&oe=UTF-8&hl=en-us&client=safari

Chemotherapy
- **Types of Chemotherapy**
  https://www.cancer.org/cancer/prostate-cancer/treating/chemotherapy.html
- **Side Effects of Chemotherapy**
  https://www.pcf.org/about-prostate-cancer/prostate-cancer-side effects/?gclid=CjwKCAjw7LX0BRBiEiwA_gNw1YyXOpAOiQGopDRO4LlUx9XAC_XL6k-tzDxlRgewfq3ASpf7FkenRoCU3oQAvD_BwE

III. Sexual Dysfunction

- **Rehabilitation of Penis After Prostate Surgery**
  https://www.health.harvard.edu/mens-health/penile-rehabilitation-after-prostate-cancer-surgery

IV. After Surgery Care

- **Blog Recovery Insights**
  https://www.google.com/search?q=home+recovery+after+surgery+blog&ie=UTF-8&oe=UTF-8&hl=en-us&client=safari

V. Complications/Pain

- **Pain Management**
  https://www.ncbi.nlm.nih.gov/pmc/articles/PMC4632348/
- **Prostate Treatment Side Effects**
  http://www.seattlecca.org/diseases/prostate-cancer/treatment-options/potential-side effects
- **Treatment of Prostate Cancer That Does Not Go Away**
  https://www.cancer.org/cancer/prostate-cancer/treating/recurrence.html
- **Surgery Complications: What patients should know**
  https://www.mskcc.org/blog/prostate-surgery-complications-what-patients-should-know
- **Groin Pain**
  https://www.cancerforums.net/threads/43373-Groin-pain-one-year-after-prostate-cancer-surgery

- **Fungus on Penis and Scrotum**
  https://www.webmd.com/skin-problems-and-treatments/guide/fungal-infections-skin
- **Penis/Scrotum Ointment Treatments**
  https://www.webmd.com/drugs/2/drug-4316/clotrimazole-topical/details
- **Yeast Infection or Diaper Rash**
  https://www.healthline.com/health/parenting/yeast-diaper-rash
- **Adult Diaper Rash**
  https://www.healthline.com/health/adult-diaper-rash

VI. Caregivers

- **Caregiver's Guide**
  https://www.urologyhealth.org/caregiverguide/
- **For Caregivers**
  https://www.dana-farber.org/health-library/articles/for-caregivers/

VII. PC Blogs, Chats, Forum Sites, and Books

- **Ten Best Cancer Blogs**
  https://www.medicalnewstoday.com/articles/318670.php
- **Personal Reflection Blogs**
  https://blog.livestrong.org/my-cancer-journey-at-five-years-a-personal-reflection-278aa8510304
- **Writing about Your Cancer Experience**

https://www.cancer.net/blog/2017-06/3-tips-writing-about-your-cancer-experience

- **My Cancer Blog**
  https://mdbcancerjourney.com/
- **About Cancer Chat**
  https://www.cancerresearchuk.org/about-cancer/cancer-chat/thread/husband-cancer
- **8 Best Prostate Cancer Forums**
  https://www.healthline.com/health/prostate-cancer/prostate-cancer-forums
- *100 Question & Answers About Prostate Cancer*
  https://www.amazon.com/Questions-Answers-About-Prostate-Cancer/dp/1284152340

Receiving a prostate cancer diagnosis is a difficult experience, and leaves patients and their caregivers feeling anxious and overwhelmed. What is prostate cancer? What are the treatment options? What are the sources of support? The only text to provide both the doctor's and patient's point of view, 100 Questions & Answers About Prostate Cancer, Fifth Edition provides authoritative, practical answers to these questions, and many more. This updated Fifth Edition provides a comprehensive discussion of what you can expect post-diagnosis along with patient commentary to give you a real-life understanding of what these steps might mean for your day-to day life. This book is an invaluable resource for anyone coping with the uncertainty of a prostate cancer diagnosis.[2]

---

[2] *100 Questions & Answers About Prostate Cancer*, Amazon.com, accessed September 20, 2022, https://www.amazon.com/Questions-Answers-About-Prostate-Cancer/dp/1284152340.

BIBLIOGRAPHY

100 Questions & Answers About Prostate Cancer. Amazon.com. Accessed September 20, 2022. https://www.amazon.com/ Questions-Answers-About-Prostate-Cancer/dp/1284152340.

Bonn, Stephanie E., Arvid Sjölander, Ylva Trolle Lagerros, Fredrik Wiklund, Pär Stattin, Erik Holmberg, Henrik Grönberg, and Katarina Bälter. "Physical activity and survival among men diagnosed with prostate cancer." *Cancer Epidemiology, Biomarkers & Prevention* 24, no. 1 (January 1, 2015): 57–64. https://doi.org/10.1158/1055-9965. EPI-14-0707.

Printed in the United States
by Baker & Taylor Publisher Services